西安交通大学"十三五"规划教材

组织学彩色图谱

Color Atlas of Histology

主编 周劲松

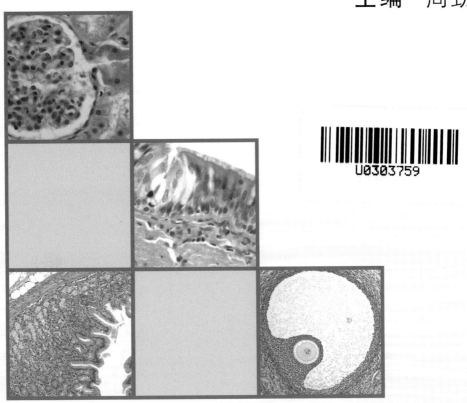

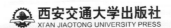
西安交通大学出版社
XI'AN JIAOTONG UNIVERSITY PRESS

图书在版编目(CIP)数据

组织学彩色图谱＝Color Atlas of Histology:汉英对照/
周劲松主编. —西安:西安交通大学出版社,2018.3
西安交通大学"十三五"规划教材
ISBN 978－7－5693－0508－1

Ⅰ.①组…　Ⅱ.①周…　Ⅲ.①人体组织学-图谱
Ⅳ.①R329－64

中国版本图书馆 CIP 数据核字(2018)第 059624 号

书　　名	组织学彩色图谱
主　　编	周劲松
责任编辑	杜玄静

出版发行	西安交通大学出版社
	(西安市兴庆南路 10 号　邮政编码 710049)
网　　址	http://www.xjtupress.com
电　　话	(029)82668357　82667874(发行中心)
	(029)82668315(总编办)
传　　真	(029)82668280
印　　刷	陕西龙山海天艺术印务有限公司

开　　本	889mm×1194mm　1/16　　**印张** 8.75　　**字数** 259 千字
版次印次	2018 年 7 月第 1 版　　2018 年 8 月第 1 次印刷
书　　号	ISBN 978－7－5693－0508－1
定　　价	46.00 元

读者购书、书店添货,如发现印装质量问题,请与本社发行中心联系、调换。
订购热线:(029)82665248　(029)82665249
投稿热线:(029)82668526　(029)82668133
读者信箱:xj_rwjg@126.com

主　审:宋天保　西安交通大学医学部
　　　　　　　　Xi'an Jiaotong University Health Science Center
主　编:周劲松　西安交通大学医学部
副主编:张晓田　西安交通大学医学部
　　　　许　颖　西安交通大学外国语学院
　　　　　　　　School of Foreign Studies，Xi'an Jiaotong University
　　　　寇　博　西安交通大学医学部第一附属医院
　　　　　　　　First Affiliated Hospital，Xi'an Jiaotong University Health Science
　　　　　　　　Center
参　编:田　宏　西安交通大学医学部
　　　　路　明　西安交通大学医学部
　　　　李媛洁　西安交通大学医学部
　　　　武　捷　西安交通大学医学部
　　　　胡海波　西安交通大学医学部
　　　　霍涌玮　西安交通大学医学部
　　　　吴晓林　西安交通大学医学部
　　　　张建水　西安交通大学医学部
　　　　冯改丰　西安交通大学医学部
　　　　许杰华　西安交通大学医学部
　　　　董炜疆　西安交通大学医学部
　　　　王　蕊　西安交通大学医学部
　　　　张　翀　西北政法大学人事处
　　　　　　　　Human Resources，Northwest University of Political Science and Law
　　　　边文博　华为技术运营商网络投标部
　　　　　　　　Carrier BG Network Bidding Dept.，Huawei Technologies
　　　　周泓成　长安大学信息工程学院
　　　　　　　　School of Information Engineering，Chang'an University
　　　　王鹤扬　西安交通大学机械工程学院
　　　　　　　　School of Mechanical Engineering，Xi'an Jiaotong University

序　言

　　组织学与胚胎学是医学生学习的一门重要基础课。除了大量的理论知识外,在实验课中还要复习、记忆、讨论和理解人体组织器官的微细结构和相关功能,为以后学习病理学、生理学和病理生理学等其他医学课程打下坚实基础。

　　在多年教学过程中,我们发现因为组织切片不同批次和质量等问题,学生在实验课上观察到的微细结构并不能完全验证理论知识,也不能完全覆盖理论课中的重点和难点。在学校、组织学专家和同事等多方支持和鼓励下,我们从科室的切片库中精挑细选,并不断制备和补充新的组织切片,历经4年,终于建立了比较健全的组织学光学显微镜电子图库。本教材从图库中选择了组织学理论教学和实验观察中的重点和难点,共计213张(图注只显示物镜放大倍数,目镜放大倍数均为10倍),能更好地帮助学生学习和理解组织学理论知识和实验技术。因篇幅限制,本教材未讨论相关功能和电镜结构,这些内容可在实验教学中讨论完成。

　　本教材适用于生物医学、基础医学、临床医学、预防医学、法医学、口腔医学和护理专业等本科和研究生学习使用,也可作为医学研究工作者参阅使用。

　　衷心感谢宋天保教授通读整本教材,在图片选择、专业术语、文字内容和写作编排等方面给予的指导。感谢本科室实验技术人员李明和王丽蓉在切片制作和显微摄影中的无私帮助。感谢编委家属对本教材编写工作的理解与支持,感谢西安交通大学出版社编辑杜玄静热忱专业的出版服务。感谢西安交通大学教务处的资助(西安交通大学"十三五"规化教材),使得本书得以顺利出版。

　　书中难免有疏漏之处,请读者不吝批评指正。

西安交通大学医学部

周劲松

2018 年 3 月

Preface

Histology and Embryology is an important basic course for medical students. Beside the lecture knowledge, the students must go over, memorize, discuss and understand numerous microstructures and corresponding functions of tissues and organs of human body in the lab to ensure that they totally master the course knowledge, and will be prepared to study other medical courses in the future, such as Pathology, Physiology and Pathophysiology, etc.

In the past decades of teaching, we found that the microstructures observed in Histology lab can not completely demonstrate the knowledge or fully cover the important and key information learnt in Histology lectures, due to the different slide batches and quality. Thus, encouraged and supported by colleges, Histology expertise and the University, we spent about 4 years to select excellent Histology slides from department slide bank, prepared new Histology slides, and finally established a relatively intact light microscope Histology electronic atlas bank via photomicrography. This book selects 213 images from the bank (The image legend shows the objective magnification times, all the ocular magnification times are 10), which covers almost all the important and key information in Histology lecture and lab. It will greatly help students learn and understand knowledge and basic technology of Histology. Due to paper limitations, the corresponding functions and electronic microscope (EM) structures are not discussed in this book, which can be studied via discussions in lab.

This textbook is suitable for undergraduate and graduate students in specialty of Biomedicine, Basic Medicine, Clinic Medicine, Preventive Medicine, Forensic medicine, Oral Medicine and Nursing, which also can be used as references for medical researchers.

We sincerely thank Professor Tianbao Song, who critically read the entire book and gave us important suggestions on image selection, Histology terminology, text and writing pattern. We thank Ming Li and Lirong Wang, the department technicians, for their selfless help in slide preparation and photomicrography. We also extend our appreciation to family members of authors for their understanding and support for compiling work, and Xuanjing Du, the staff of Xi'an Jiaotong Universiy Press, for her editorial enthusiasm and expertise. We thank Dean's Office of Xi'an Jiaotong University who gave us financial support for the publishing the Thirteenth Five-year Plan programming textbook, Xi'an Jiaotong University.

Oversights and deficiencies may appear in the book, any corrections and suggestions are greatly appreciated.

Jinsong Zhou, PhD
Health Science Center
Xi'an Jiaotong University
March, 2018

目　录
catalogue

第一章　组织学标本制作和常用染色方法

一、组织学标本的制作

大部分组织学标本来源于人体,但也可来源于兔、猫、鼠、狗、羊和猪等动物,因其取材更加方便。取材时需要迅速精准而轻微,避免组织腐败或受损。

1.固定:目的是将蛋白质等变性,尽量保持组织结构和成分与其存活状态时类似。大部分固定剂的溶剂是水。

2.脱水、透明和包埋:通常用浓度梯度上升酒精等脱水剂将固定后组织中的水分完全置换,用二甲苯等透明剂将脱水剂完全置换,再用 $56\sim60$ ℃的液态石蜡等包埋剂完全置换透明剂。在室温时石蜡凝固,组织即成硬化的固态,利于切片。

3.切片:用石蜡切片机或冷冻切片机等将组织块切成 7 μm 厚的组织切片,该厚度相当于人体细胞平均直径,能保障染料着色充分又利于观察时清晰聚焦。若组织为薄膜状,可制备组织铺片;如组织坚固,可制备组织磨片;如组织为液态,可制备涂片;必要时可将软化的组织块制成压片。

4.裱片:用涂有黏附剂的洁净载玻片捞取温水表面漂浮的石蜡切片,或沾取冷冻切片机制备的冷冻切片。

5.脱蜡:用二甲苯处理石蜡切片以除去石蜡,再经浓度梯度下降酒精处理入水,因染料常为水溶性。

二、常用染色方法

染色的目的是改变组织切片中不同结构的折光率,增加其光学对比性。组织学最常用的染料是苏木素和伊红,用它们来染色的方法称为苏木素-伊红(HE)染色。还可用甲苯胺蓝、银盐染色或 Wright's 染色法等。在研究组织中的化学成分时,PAS 反应、福尔根反应和四氧化锇可分别显示多糖、核酸和脂类;四唑盐法和 TUNEL 染色分别显示脱氢酶和细胞凋亡;免疫组织化学和原位杂交能分别精确地显示各类蛋白质和特定核苷酸序列的核酸片段。

1.HE 染色:苏木精(hematoxylin)是碱性化学物质,为蓝紫色染料,被苏木精着色的结构称嗜碱性结构;伊红(eosin)是酸性化学物质,为红色染料,被伊红着色的结构称嗜酸性结构;少数结构对苏木精或伊红均不敏感,称中性。

2.过碘酸希夫(periodic acid Schiff,PAS)反应:是组织化学中显示多糖的方法之一。其原理是用过碘酸将糖分子中的 1,2-二醇基氧化成游离二醛基,再用无色亚硫酸品红(希夫试剂)与醛基反应,从而在原位形成紫红色沉淀。

3.福尔根反应(Feulgen reaction):是组织化学中显示 DNA 的方法之一。其原理是用稀盐酸水解DNA,打开嘌呤碱基与脱氧核糖之间的糖苷键,形成醛基,再与希夫试剂反应,从而在原位形成紫红色沉淀。

4.酶组织化学染色:酶是有催化功能的蛋白质,如乳酸脱氢酶。在特定条件下,乳酸脱氢酶将底物乳酸转变为丙酮酸,释放的氢将无色的氮蓝四唑(NBT)转变为蓝色沉淀。

5.免疫组织化学染色:在免疫组织化学染色中,将待探测的蛋白质作为抗原,利用抗原-抗体反应,最终将带有荧光或其他标记的抗体原位结合于抗原处,再显示标记,从而显示抗原。

6.原位末端标记法(TUNEL 染色):细胞凋亡是程序性死亡,在凋亡的过程中细胞仍然有新陈代谢,但凋亡细胞的 DNA 双链会断裂或一条链出现缺口,产生一系列 3'-OH 末端。TUNEL 染色法中,在脱氧核糖核苷酸末端转移酶作用下,将生物素等标记的 dUTP 连接到 3'-OH 末端,再通过组化或免疫组化等方法显示生物素,形成棕色沉淀。

染色后的标本经上升酒精脱水,二甲苯透明,滴加中性树胶后,盖玻片封固,称干封法。对于溶于酒精或二甲苯的染料或不能长期保存的染色,可滴加缓冲液等湿封短期保存。干封保存时间长久,因中性树胶折光率高而成像更清晰。

注意:制备组织标本过程中,会出现因人工操作不当而造成的结构假象,如组织脱落、脱水或透明不彻底、标本有刀痕、折叠或污染、染色不均或褪色以及组织自溶等。观察组织结构时需注意辨别。

Chapter 1   Commonly used methods in tissue preparation and staining

Ⅰ. Procedure for tissue preparation

Most specimens come from human body while some are from rabbit, cat, rat, dog, goat and pig, etc, because it is more convenient to obtain specimens from animals than from human being. The specimen collection must be rapid, accurate and gentle to avoid the decay and damages to tissue.

1 **Fixation**   Fixatives are introduced to denature tissue proteins and preserve tissue structures as possible as it can. Water is the solvent of most fixatives.

2 **Dehydration, clearing and embedding**   Usually, the concentration gradient ascending alcohol is used to totally replace water in tissue after fixation, and the xylene thoroughly replaces the alcohol. At $56\sim60℃$, the melted paraffin replaces xylene and the tissue block becomes solid at room temperature for sectioning.

3 **Sectioning**   Usually the regular or freezing microtome is used to cut the tissue block into 7-μm-thick sections, which is the average diameter of human body cells. The section containing 1 layer of the cells guarantees better staining, and is easy to be focused under microscope. The stretched preparation for membrane tissue, ground section for hard tissue, smear for fluid tissue and tableting for softened tissue are also common section methods.

4 **Adherence**   Glue-coated glass slides are used to attach the paraffin sections on the surface of warm water or the frozen sections in freezing microtome.

5 **Dewaxing**   The paraffin sections are treated by xylene to remove paraffin and then by concentration gradientdescending alcohol to water, because the dyes are usually water soluble.

Ⅱ. Commonly used staining methods

The purpose of staining is to change the refractive indices of different structures in sections and increase the optical contrast. The commonly used dyes in Histology are hematoxylin (H) and eosin (E), and the staining method using H and E is called HE staining. Toluidine blue, silver salts and Wright's staining can also be introduced. When studying tissue chemical compositions, PAS reaction, Feulgen reaction and OsO_4 are used to show polysaccharides, nucleic acids and lipids, respectively. Tetrazolium and TUNEL staining are used to demonstrate dehydrogenase and cell apoptosis, respectively. Immunohistochemical staining and in situ hybridization are introduced to detect proteins and nucleic acid fragments containing specific sequence of nucleotides, respectively.

1 **Hematoxylin-eosin staining**   Hematoxylin is a basic blue dye, and the structure stained by hematox-

ylin is called basophilic structure. Eosin is an acid pink dye, and the structure stained by eosin is called acidophilic structure. Some structures are known as neutrophilic structures because they are insensitive to either hematoxylin or eosin.

2　**Periodic acid Schiff (PAS) reaction**　PAS reaction is designed to detect polysaccharides in histochemistry. The periodic acid is used to oxidize 1,2-glycol groups in the sugar molecules into free aldehyde groups, which then react with colorless sulphurous acid fuchsin (Schiff reagent) to form magenta deposit.

3　**Feulgen reaction**　Feulgen reaction is designed to detect DNA in histochemistry. The mild hydrochloric acid is used to cleave the glycosidic bonds between purine bases and deoxyribose to form aldehyde groups, which then react with Schiff reagent to form magenta deposits.

4　**Enzyme histochemistry**　Enzymes are the proteins with catalytic power, such as lactate dehydrogenase (LDH). LDH catalyzes lactic acid into pyruvic acid under specific conditions and the released hydrogen combines with the nitroblue tetrazolium (NBT) to form blue deposits.

5　**Immunohistochemistry**　In the immunohistochemical staining, the detected proteins are regarded as antigens, and the antibodies conjugated with fluorescence dye or other markers combine with antigens in situ, and then the markers are visualized.

6　**Terminal deoxynucleotidyl transferase-mediated dUTP nick end labeling (TUNEL)**　Apoptosis is programmed cell death, during which the cells still metabolize. While cells undergo apoptosis, the DNA double-strands fracture or a single-strand breaks, resulting in a series of $3'$-OH ends. With TUNEL staining, biotin labeled-dUTP are linked to $3'$-OH ends by terminal deoxyribonucleotidyl transferase and then visualized by histochemical or immunohistochemical method.

Reservation: In the dry reservation, the sections undergo dehydration by ascending alcohol and clearance by xylene, and then are immersed in neutral balsam and covered by cover slips. In some cases, the final color can not tolerate alcohol or xylene, or the color fades quickly, so the sections have to be immersed in buffer for wet reservation for short term. The dry reservation keeps sections more clearly for a long time because the neutral balsam is highly refractive.

Artifacts may occur during tissue preparation, such as tissue shedding from the slide, incomplete dehydration or clearance, knife scratch, folding or contamination in tissue sections, nonuniform staining or color fading, and tissue autolysis, etc. These artifacts must be distinguished from normal structures.

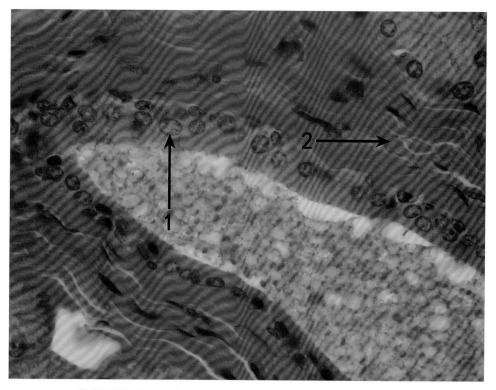

1. 嗜碱性结构(basophilic structure) 2. 嗜酸性结构(acidophilic structure)

图 1-1 下颌下腺:人(HE 染色,×100)

Pic. 1-1 Submandibular gland:Human. HE staining ×100

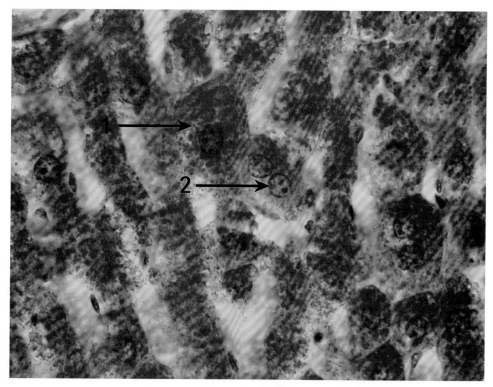

1. 胞质糖原(glycogens in cytoplasm) 2. 肝细胞核(nucleus of a hepatocyte)

图 1-2 肝脏:人(PAS反应,×100)

Pic. 1-2 Liver:Human. PAS reaction ×100

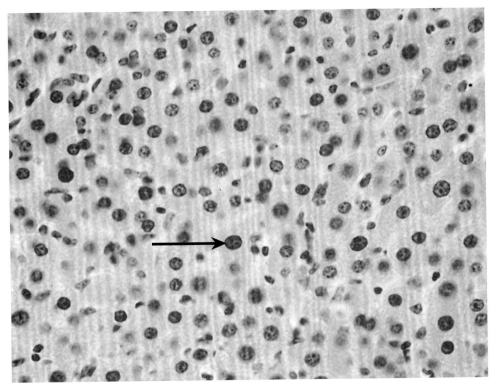

箭头示细胞核中的 DNA。The arrow shows DNA in nucleus.

图 1 - 3 肝脏:人(Feulgen 反应,×20)

Pic. 1 - 3 Liver:Human. Feulgen reaction ×20

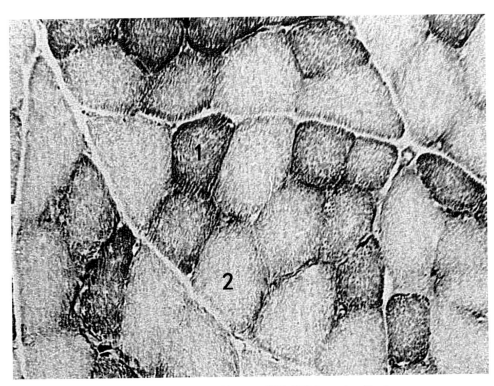

1.阳性纤维(positive fiber) 2.阴性纤维(negative fiber)

图 1 - 4 骨骼肌:人(乳酸脱氢酶组织化学染色,×40)

Pic. 1 - 4 Skeletal muscle:Human. Lactic dehydrogenase histochemical staining ×40

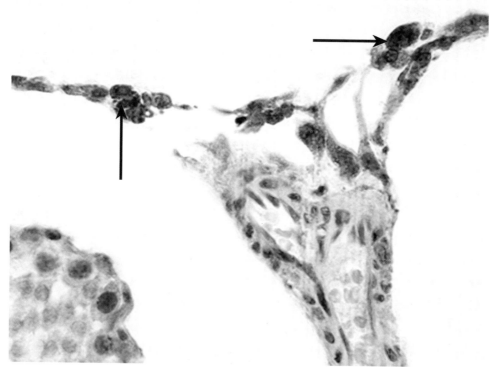

箭头示间质细胞棕色胞质含 P 物质样物质。

The brown Leydig cell cytoplasm marked by arrows indicates that there are Substance P-like substance.

图 1－5　睾丸：大鼠（免疫酶染色，DAB 显色，×40）

Pic. 1－5　Testis：Rat. Immunoenzyme staining，DAB visualization　×40

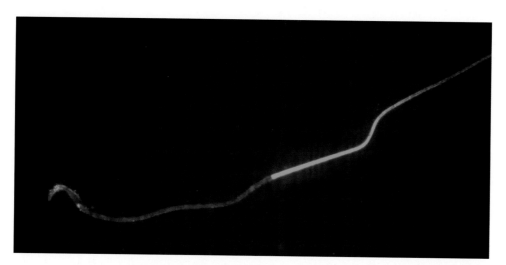

精子尾部亮绿色示其含精子相关抗原样物质。

The bright green color of the tail shows that it contains Sperm associated antigen11C-like substance.

图 1－6　精子：小鼠（免疫荧光染色，×40）

Pic. 1－6　Spermato zoon：Mouse. Immunofluorescence staining　×40

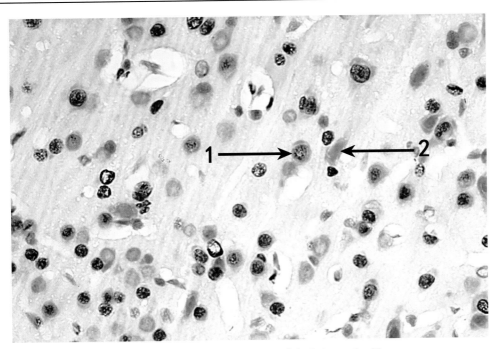

1.凋亡细胞(apoptotic cell)　2.正常细胞(normal cell)

图 1 - 7　脑:兔(TUNEL 染色,×40)

Pic. 1 - 7　Brain:Rabbit. TUNEL staining　×40

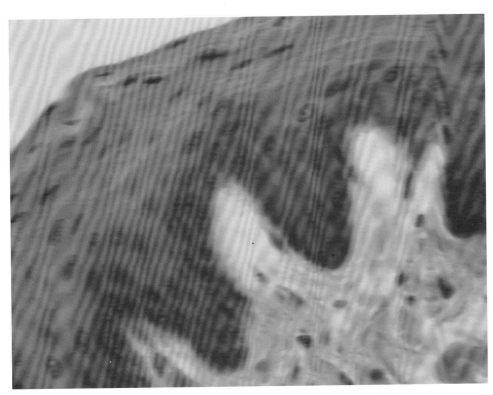

结构模糊提示染色后封存时脱水透明不彻底。此为人工假象。

The obscure structure suggests that the dehydration and clearance are not thorough after staining. It is an artifact.

图 1 - 8　舌:猫(HE 染色,×40)

Pic. 1 - 8　Tongue:Cat. HE staining　×40

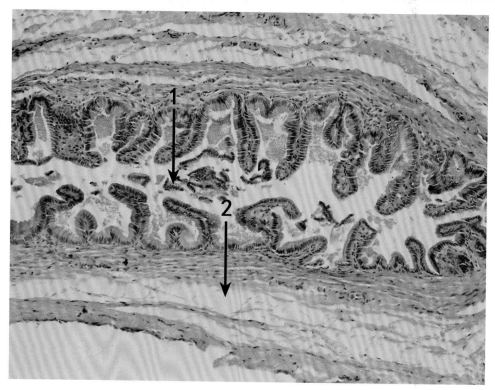

1.脱落结构(shedding structure) 2.组织制备造成的裂隙(tissue fissure caused by sample preparation) 均为人工假象。These are artifacts.

图 1-9 胆囊：人(HE 染色，×20)

Pic. 1-9 Gall bladder：Human. HE staining ×20

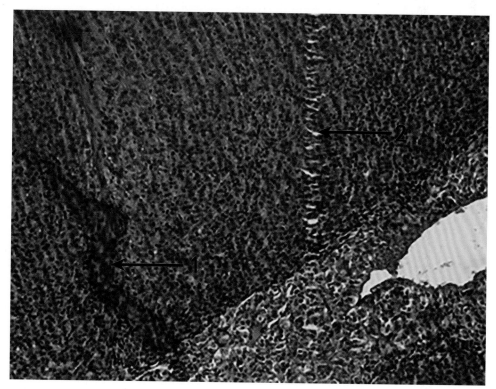

1.组织折叠(tissue folding) 2.组织划痕(knife scratch) 均为人工假象。These are artifacts.

图 1-10 肾上腺：兔(HE 染色，×40)

Pic. 1-10 Adrenal gland：Rabbit. HE staining ×40

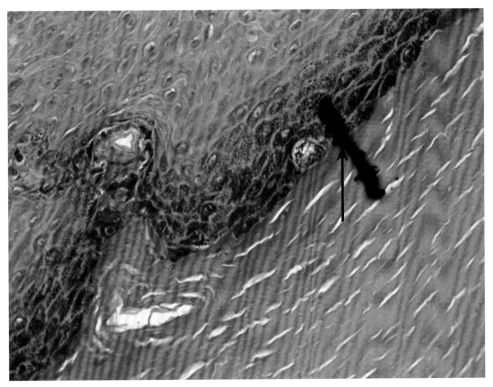

箭头示污染物。此为人工假象。The arrow shows the contaminant. This is an artifact.

图 1-11 指皮：人（HE 染色，×40）

Pic. 1-11 Finger skin：Human. HE staining ×40

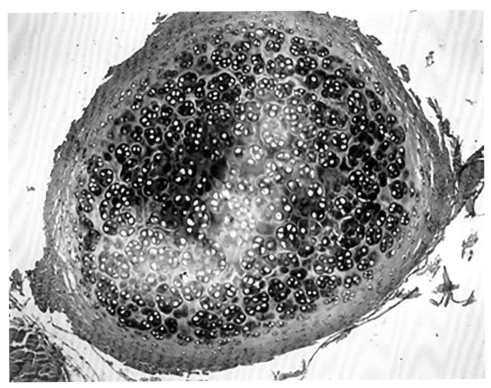

染色不均。此为人工假象。Unbalanced staining. This is an artifact.

图 1-12 肋软骨：兔（HE 染色，×10）

Pic. 1-12 Costal cartilage：Rabbit. HE staining ×10

第二章　上皮组织

实验基本要求：

1. 了解腺体的分类。多细胞外分泌腺的结构和分类。

2. 熟悉蛋白质分泌细胞、糖蛋白分泌细胞和类固醇分泌细胞的光学显微镜（LM）和电镜（EM）结构特点。

3. 掌握上皮组织的分类和一般特点。单层扁平上皮、单层立方上皮、单层柱状上皮、假复层纤毛柱状上皮、复层扁平上皮和变移上皮的结构、主要分布和功能。

4. 掌握上皮组织各种特殊结构的 LM 和 EM 结构和功能：微绒毛、纤毛、紧密连接、中间连接、桥粒、缝隙连接、连接复合体、基膜、质膜内褶和半桥粒。

5. 光镜下识别单层扁平上皮、单层立方上皮、单层柱状上皮、假复层纤毛柱状上皮、复层扁平上皮和变移上皮。

6. 相关超微结构和功能可通过课堂讨论等完成。

Chapter 2　Epithelial tissue

 Basic requirements for the experiment

1. Know the classifications of gland, the structures and classifications of multi-cell exocrine glands.

2. Familiar with the structural characteristics of protein,glycoprotein and steroid-secreting cell under LM and EM.

3. Familiar with the classifications and general features of the epithelial tissues. The structures, distributions and functions of the simple squamous epithelium, simple cuboidal epithelium, simple columnar epithelium, pseudostratified ciliated columnar epithelium, stratified squamous epithelium and transitional epithelium.

4. Master the structures and functions of epithelial specializations：microvillus,cilium,tight junction,intermediate junction,desmosome,gap junction,junctional complex,basement membrane,plasma membrane infolding,hemidesmosome under LM and EM.

5. Identify simple squamous epithelium,simple cuboidal epithelium,simple columnar epithelium, pseudostratified ciliated columnar epithelium,stratified squamous epithelium and transitional epithelium under LM.

6. The corresponding EM structures and functions will be discussed in lab.

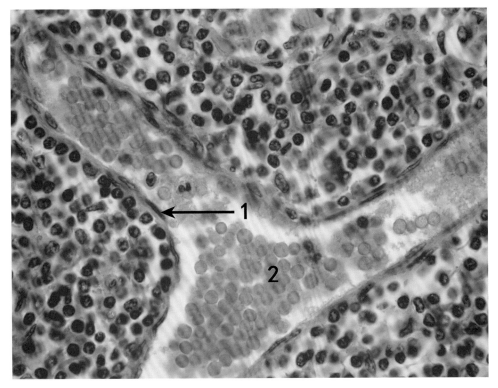

1. 内皮(endothelium)　2. 血管内的红细胞(red blood cells in a vessel)

图 2-1　内皮：狗淋巴结髓质(HE 染色，×100)

Pic. 2-1　Endothelium：Medulla of dog lymphatic node. HE staining　×100

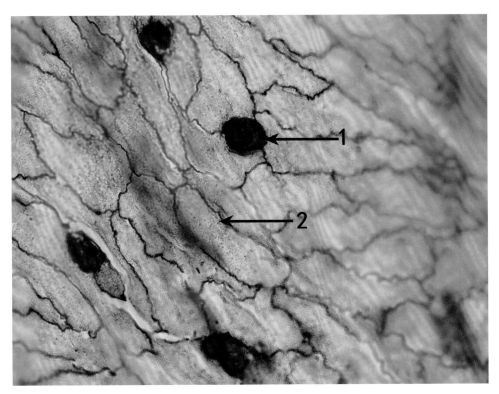

1. 间皮细胞核(nucleus of a mesothelial cell)　2. 间皮细胞边界(mesothelial cell boundary)

图 2-2　间皮：蛙腹膜(铺片，银染，×100)

Pic. 2-2　Mesothelium：Frog peritoneum. Stretched preparation. Silver staining　×100

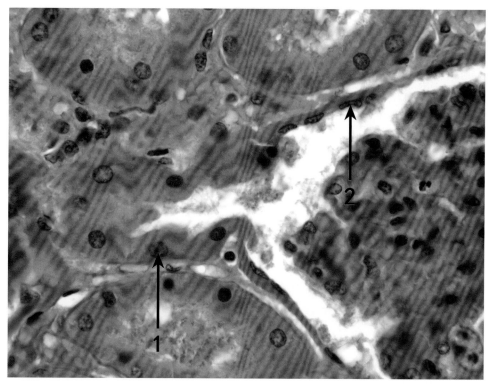

1. 单层立方上皮(simple cuboidal epithelium) 2. 单层扁平上皮(simple squamous epithelium)

图 2-3 单层扁平上皮和单层立方上皮:人肾小球(HE 染色,×100)

Pic. 2-3 Simple squamous epithelium and simple cuboidal epithelium:Glomerulus of human kidney. HE staining ×100

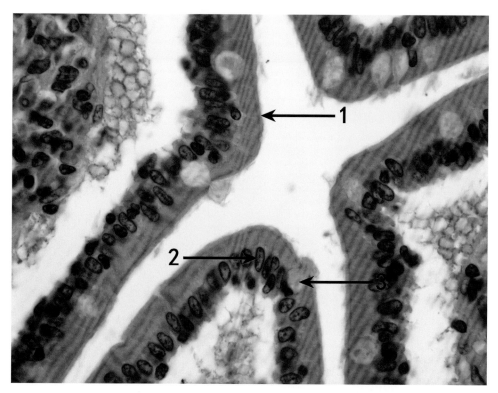

1. 纹状缘(striated border) 2. 柱状细胞(columnar cell) 3. 杯状细胞(goblet cell)

图 2-4 单层柱状上皮:猫回肠黏膜(HE 染色,×100)

Pic. 2-4 Simple columnar epithelium:Mucosa of cat ileum. HE staining ×100

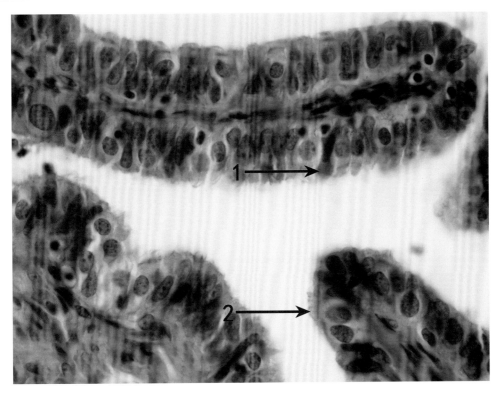

1. 分泌细胞(secretory cell) 2. 柱状细胞的纤毛(cilia of columnar cell)

图 2-5 单层纤毛柱状上皮:人输卵管黏膜(HE 染色,×100)

Pic. 2-5 Simple ciliated columnar epithelium:Mucosa of human oviduct. HE staining ×100

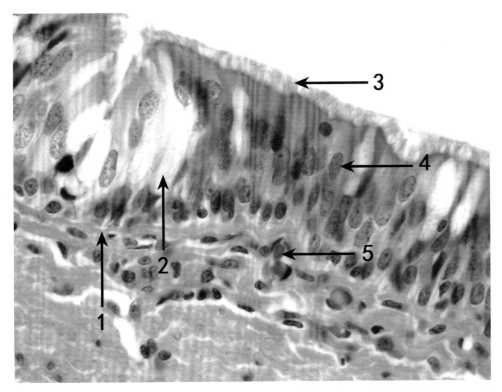

1. 基膜(basement membrane) 2. 杯状细胞(goblet cell) 3. 纤毛(cilia) 4. 柱状细胞(columnar cell)

5. 结缔组织中毛细血管(capillary in connective tissue)

图 2-6 假复层纤毛柱状上皮:人气管黏膜(HE 染色,×100)

Pic. 2-6 Pseudostratified ciliated columnar epithelium:Mucosa of human trachea. HE staining ×100

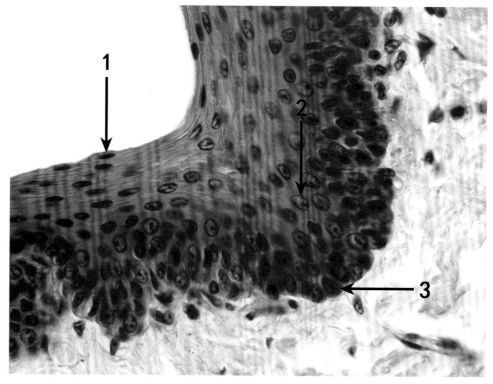

1.表层未角化细胞(nonkeratinized cell in superficial layer) 2.中间层细胞(cell in middle layer)

3.基底层细胞(cell in basal layer)

图 2-7 未角化复层扁平上皮:人食管黏膜(HE 染色,×100)

Pic. 2-7 Nonkeratinized stratified squamous epithelium:Mucosa of human esophagus. HE staining ×100

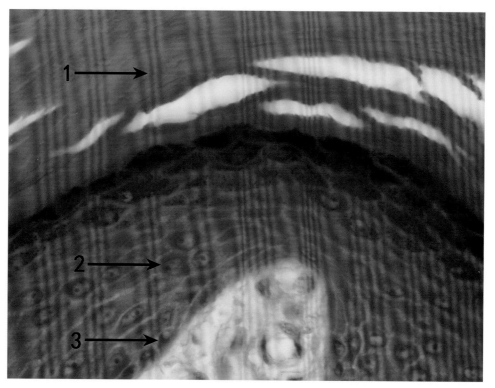

1.表层角化细胞(keratinized cell in superficial layer) 2.中间层细胞(cell in middle layer)

3.基底层细胞(cell in basal layer)

图 2-8 角化复层扁平上皮:人指皮(HE 染色,×100)

Pic. 2-8 Keratinized stratified squamous epithelium:Human finger skin. HE staining ×100

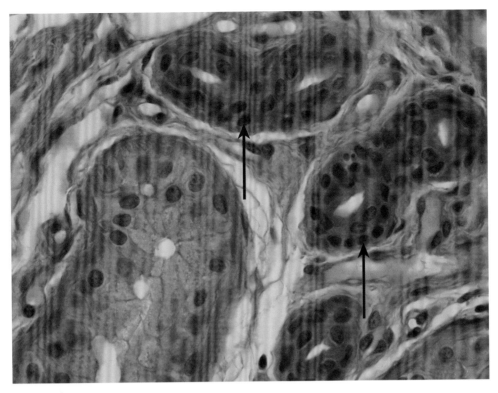

图 2-9　复层立方上皮：人指皮汗腺导管（HE 染色，×100）

Pic. 2-9　Stratified cuboidal epithelium：Human finger skin，duct of sweat gland. HE staining　×100

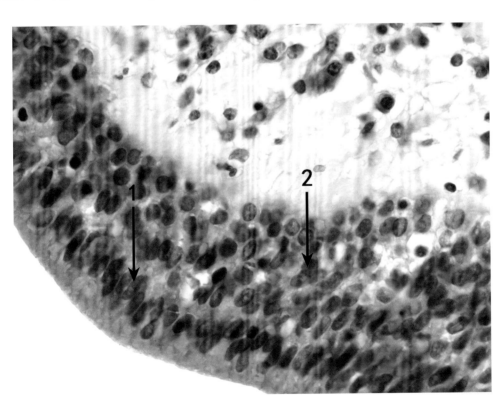

1. 表层细胞（cell in superficial layer）　2.基底层细胞（cell in basal layer）

图 2-10　复层柱状上皮：人（男）尿道黏膜（HE 染色，×100）

Pic. 2-10　Stratified columnar epithelium：Mucosa of human（male）urethra. HE staining　×100

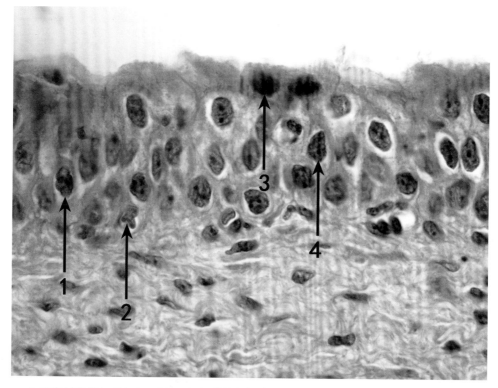

1.基底层细胞(cell in basal layer) 2.结缔组织中毛细血管(capillary in connective tissue)
3.表层细胞(cell in superficial layer) 4.中间层细胞(cell in middle layer)
图 2-11 变移上皮:猫膀胱黏膜(HE 染色,×100)
Pic. 2-11 Transitional epithelium:Mucosa of cat urinary bladder. HE staining ×100

第三章　固有结缔组织

实验基本要求：

1. 了解网状组织的结构特点和功能。

2. 了解脂肪组织、致密结缔组织的分类、结构特点和功能。

3. 熟悉结缔组织的分类和一般特点。

4. 熟悉疏松结缔组织的分布、结构特点和功能。

5. 熟悉胶原纤维、弹性纤维和网状纤维的分布、光镜结构、电镜结构、化学成分和功能。

6. 掌握成纤维细胞、巨噬细胞、浆细胞和肥大细胞的光镜结构、电镜结构和功能。

7. 光镜下识别成纤维细胞、巨噬细胞、浆细胞、肥大细胞、胶原纤维、弹性纤维、网状纤维、网状组织、脂肪组织、规则和不规则致密结缔组织。

8. 相关超微结构和功能可通过课堂讨论等完成。

Chapter 3　Connective tissue proper

 Basic requirements for the experiment

1. Know the structures and functions of reticular tissue.

2. Know the classifications, structural characteristics and functions of adipose tissue and dense connective tissue.

3. Familiar with the classifications and general features of connective tissue.

4. Familiar with the distributions, structures and functions of loose connective tissue.

5. Familiar with the distributions, LM and EM structures, chemical compositions and functions of collagenous fiber, elastic fiber and reticular fiber.

6. Master the structures and functions of fibroblast, macrophage, plasma cell and mast cell under LM and EM.

7. Identify fibroblasts, macrophage, plasma cell, mast cell, collagenous fiber, elastic fiber, reticular fiber, reticular tissue, adipose tissue and regular and irregular dense connective tissue under LM.

8. The corresponding EM structures and functions will be discussed in lab.

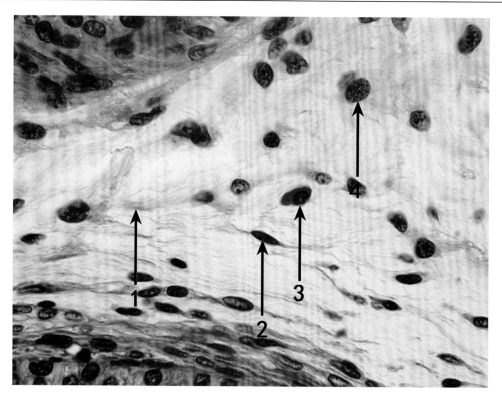

1.胶原纤维(collagenous fiber) 2.纤维细胞(fibrocyte) 3.巨噬细胞(macrophage) 4.成纤维细胞(fibroblast)

图 3-1 疏松结缔组织:人附睾(HE 染色,×100)

Pic. 3-1 Loose connective tissue:Human epididymis. HE staining ×100

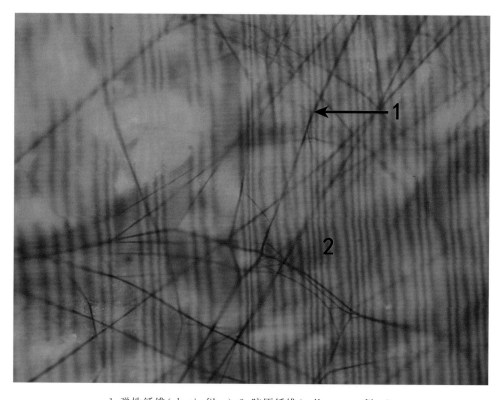

1.弹性纤维(elastic fiber) 2.胶原纤维(collagenous fiber)

图 3-2 弹性纤维:大鼠肠系膜铺片(地衣红-伊红染色,×100)

Pic. 3-2 Elastic fiber:Rat mesentery. Stretched preparation. Orcein-Eosin staining ×100

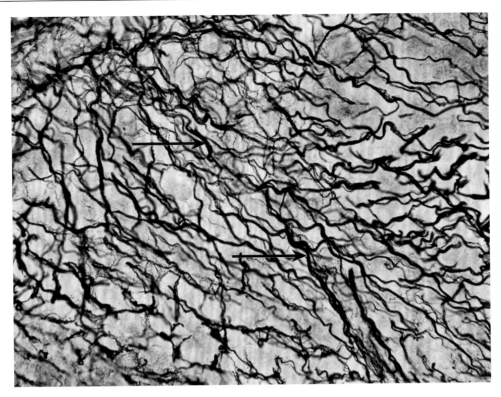

箭头示网状纤维。The arrows show reticular fibers.

图 3-3 网状组织：猫脾脏（银染，×100）

Pic. 3-3 Reticular tissue：Cat spleen. Silver staining ×100

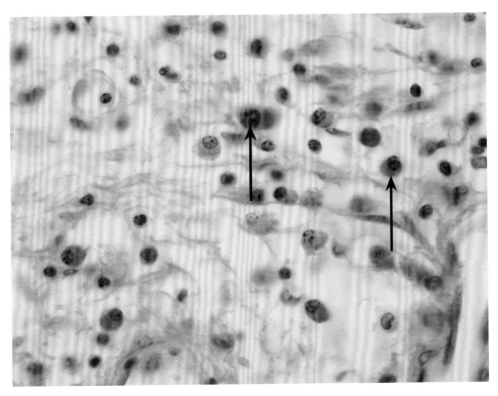

箭头示浆细胞。The arrows show plasma cells.

图 3-4 浆细胞：人鼻息肉（HE 染色，×100）

Pic. 3-4 Plasma cell：Human nasal polyp. HE staining ×100

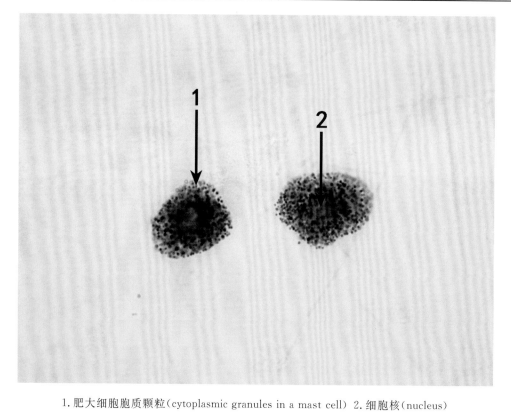

1.肥大细胞胞质颗粒(cytoplasmic granules in a mast cell) 2.细胞核(nucleus)

图 3 - 5 肥大细胞:大鼠肠系膜铺片(甲苯胺蓝染色,×100)

Pic. 3 - 5 Mast cell:Rat mesentery. Stretched preparation. Toluidine blue staining ×100

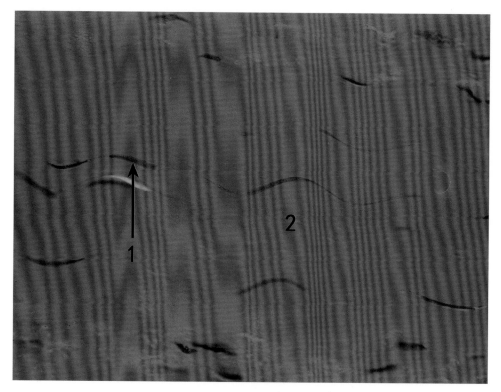

1.腱细胞(tendon cell) 2.平行排列的胶原纤维束(parallelly arranged collagen fiber)

图 3 - 6 规则致密结缔组织:人肌腱(HE 染色,×100)

Pic. 3 - 6 Regular dense connective tissue:Human tendon. HE staining ×100

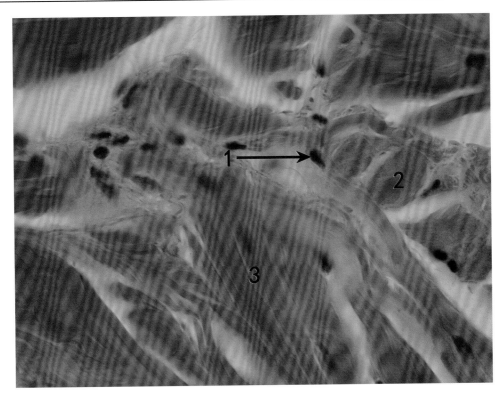

1.成纤维细胞(fibroblast) 2 和 3.纵横交错的胶原纤维束(collagenous fibers bundle in different directions)

图 3-7 不规则致密结缔组织:人真皮(HE 染色,×100)

Pic. 3-7 Irregular dense connective tissue:Human dermis. HE staining ×100

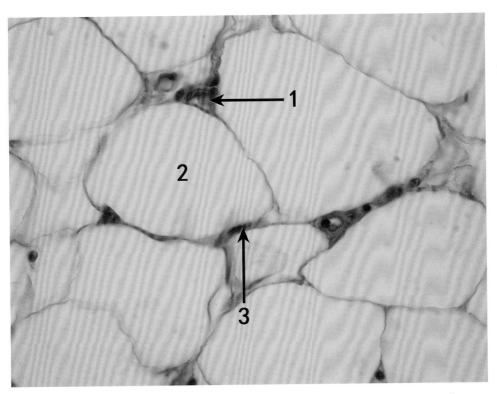

1.毛细血管(capillary) 2.单个大脂滴(已溶掉)[single big drop of lipid(dissolved)]

3.脂肪细胞的细胞核(nucleus of an adipocyte)

图 3-8 黄色脂肪组织:人肠壁(HE 染色,×100)

Pic. 3-8 Yellow adipose tissue:Human intestinal wall. HE staining ×100

第四章　软骨和骨

实验基本要求：

1. 了解软骨组织的一般结构特点和分类。

2. 了解膜内成骨和软骨内成骨的主要过程。

3. 熟悉纤维软骨和弹性软骨的分布、结构和功能。

4. 掌握透明软骨的分布、结构和功能。软骨膜的结构和功能。

5. 掌握骨板、成骨细胞、骨细胞和破骨细胞的 LM 和 EM 结构及功能。

6. 掌握环骨板、骨单位、间骨板、骨松质、骨内、外膜的结构与功能。

7. 光镜下识别透明软骨、纤维软骨、弹性软骨、骨板、成骨细胞、破骨细胞、环骨板、骨单位、间骨板和骨松质。

8. 相关超微结构和功能可通过课堂讨论等完成。

Chapter 4　Cartilage and bone

 Basic requirements for the experiment

1. Know the general features and classifications of cartilage tissue.

2. Know the processes of intramembranous ossification and endochondral ossification.

3. Familiar with the distributions, structures and functions of fibrocartilage and elastic cartilage.

4. Master the distributions, structures and functions of hyaline cartilage. The structures and functions of perichondrium.

5. Master the LM and EM structures and functions of bone lamella, osteoblast, osteocyte and osteoclast.

6. Master the structures and functions of circumferential lamella, osteon, interstitial lamella, spongy bone, endosteum and periosteum.

7. Identify hyaline cartilage, fibrocartilage, elastic cartilage, bone lamella, osteoblast, osteoclast, circumferential lamella, osteon, interstitial lamella and spongy bone under LM.

8. The corresponding EM structures and functions will be discussed in lab.

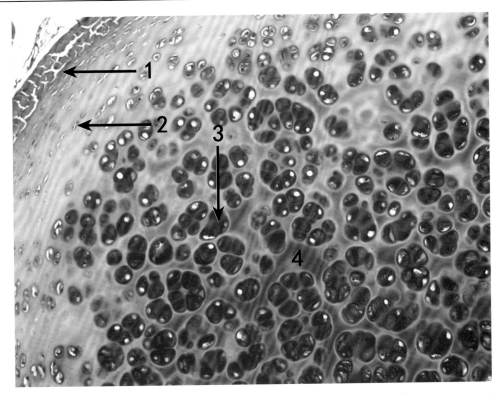

1. 软骨膜(perichondrium) 2. 幼稚软骨细胞(young chondrocyte) 3. 同源细胞群(isogenous group)
4. 软骨基质(cartilage matrix)

图 4-1 透明软骨:兔肋软骨(HE 染色,×20)

Pic. 4-1 Hyaline cartilage:Rabbit costal cartilage. HE staining ×20

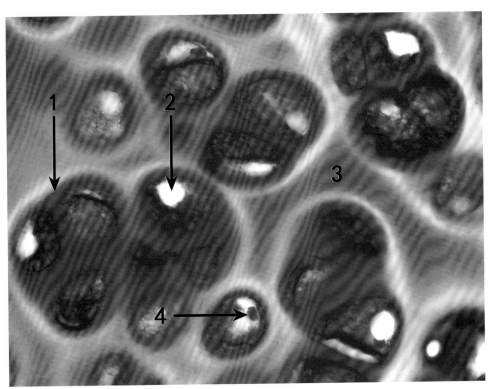

1. 软骨囊(cartilage capsule) 2. 软骨陷窝(cartilage lacuna) 3. 软骨基质(cartilage matrix) 4. 软骨细胞(chondrocyte)

图 4-2 透明软骨:兔肋软骨(HE 染色,×100)

Pic. 4-2 Hyaline cartilage:Rabbit costal cartilage. HE staining ×100

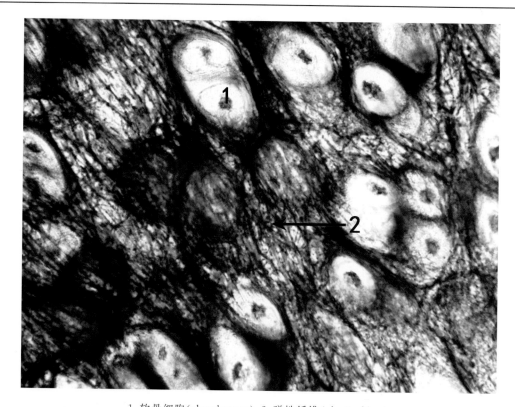

1. 软骨细胞(chondrocyte) 2. 弹性纤维(elastic fiber)
图 4 - 3 弹性软骨:人耳廓(醛复红染色, ×100)
Pic. 4 - 3 Elastic cartilage:Human auricle. Aldehyde-fuchsin staining ×100

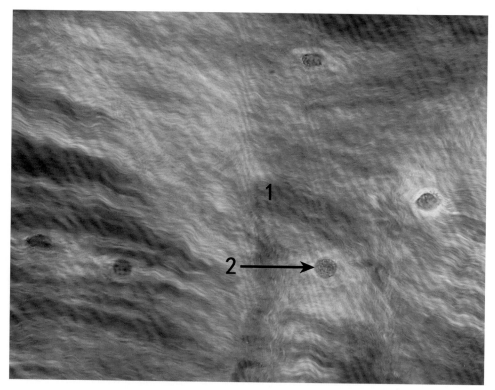

1. 胶原纤维束(collagen fiber bundle) 2. 软骨细胞(chondrocyte)
图 4 - 4 纤维软骨:人椎间盘(Mallory 三色染色, ×100)
Pic. 4 - 4 Fibrocartilage:Human intervertebral disk. Mallory trichrome staining ×100

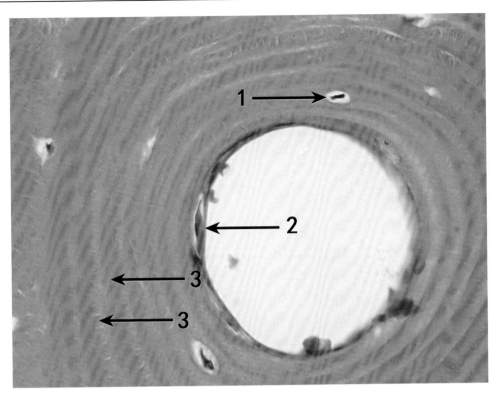

1.骨细胞(osteocyte) 2.骨内膜(endosteum) 3.骨板(bone lamellae)

图 4 - 5 骨板:人长骨(HE 染色,×100)

Pic. 4 - 5 Bone lamella:Human long bone. HE staining ×100

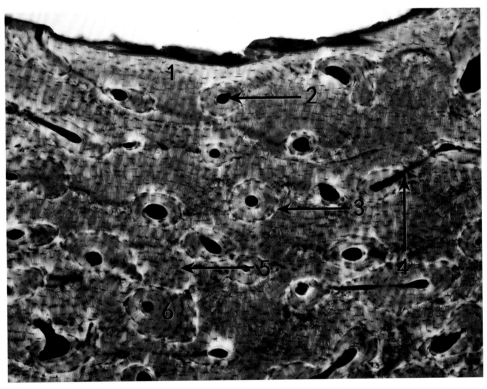

1.内环骨板(inner circumferential lamella) 2.中央管(central canal) 3.黏合线(cement line)

4.穿通管(perforating canal) 5.间骨板(interstitial lamella) 6.骨单位(osteon)

图 4 - 6 长骨:人(磨片,大丽紫染色,×10)

Pic. 4 - 6 Long bone:Human. Ground section,Dahlia violet staining ×10

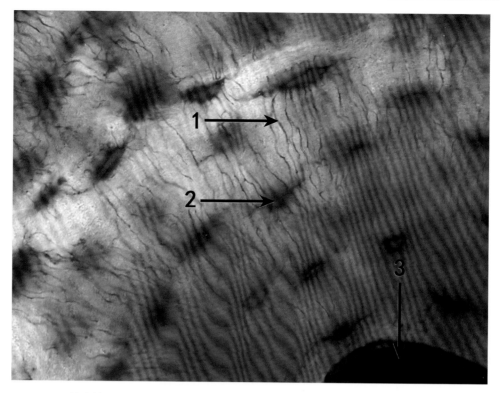

1. 骨小管（bone canaliculus） 2. 骨陷窝（bone lacuna） 3. 中央管（central canal）

图 4 - 7 骨单位：人（磨片。大丽紫染色，×100）

Pic. 4 - 7 Osteon：Human. Ground section. Dahlia violet staining ×100

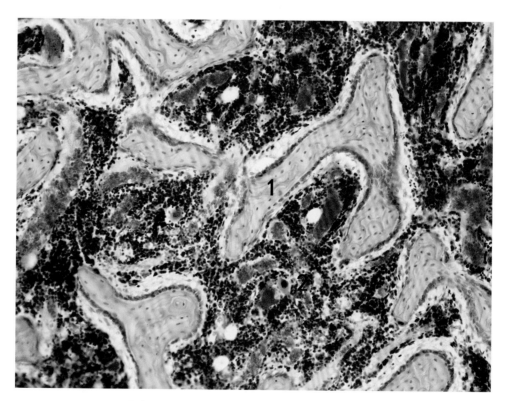

1. 骨小梁（bone trabecula） 2. 红骨髓（red bone marrow）

图 4 - 8 骨松质：人（HE 染色，×20）

Pic. 4 - 8 Spongy bone：Human. HE staining ×20

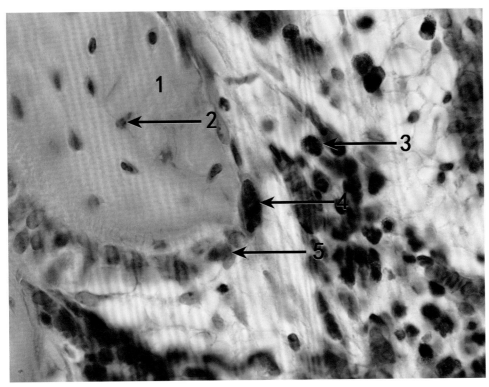

1.骨小梁(bone trabecula)　2.骨细胞(osteocyte)　3.红骨髓(red bone marrow)

4.破骨细胞(osteoclast)　5.成骨细胞(osteoblast)

图 4 - 9　骨松质:人(HE 染色,×100)

Pic. 4 - 9　Spongy bone:Human. HE staining　×100

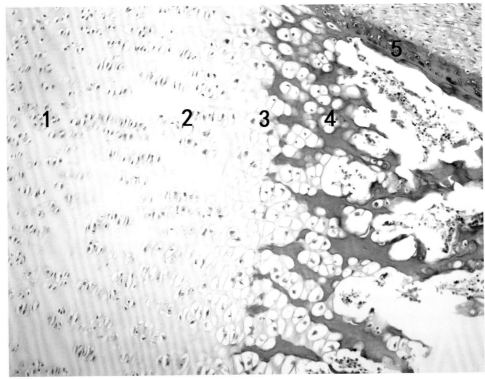

1.软骨储备区(reserve cartilage zone)　2.软骨增生区(proliferating cartilage zone)

3.软骨成熟区(maturing cartilage zone)　4.软骨钙化区(calcified cartilage zone)　5.成骨区(ossification zone)

图 4 - 10　软骨内成骨:胎儿指骨(HE 染色,×10)

Pic. 4 - 10　Endochondral ossification:Fetal phalanx. HE staining　×10

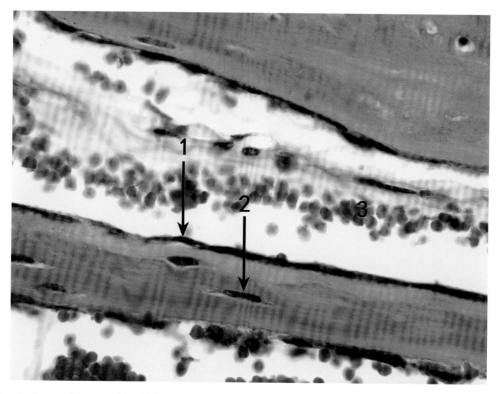

1. 成骨细胞(osteoblast) 2. 骨小梁内的骨细胞(osteocyte in bone trabecula) 3. 骨髓腔(bone marrow cavity)

图 4 - 11　膜内成骨:胎儿顶骨(HE 染色,×100)

Pic. 4 - 11　Intramembranous ossification:Fetal parietal bone. HE staining　×100

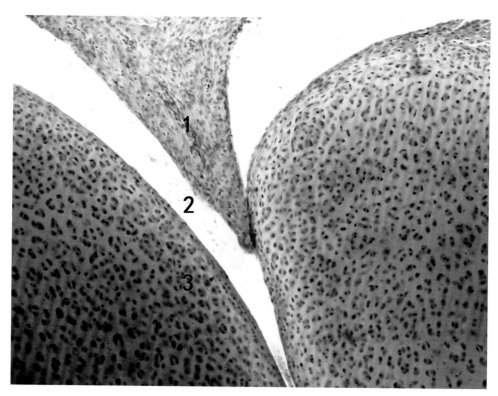

1. 滑膜(synovial membrane) 2. 关节腔(joint cavity) 3. 关节软骨(articular cartilage)

图 4 - 12　滑膜关节:胎儿指骨(HE 染色,×10)

Pic. 4 - 12　Synovial joint:Fetal phalanx. HE staining　×10

第五章　血　液

实验基本要求：

1.了解油镜的使用方法。

2.了解骨髓的组织结构。

3.熟悉血液的组成和血细胞的分类。

4.掌握红细胞的大小、形态、结构和功能。红细胞、血红蛋白、网织红细胞的正常值。

5.掌握白细胞的分类和正常值。各类白细胞的形态、结构、百分数和功能。

6.掌握血小板的形态、结构、正常值和功能。

7.油镜下掌握并识别各种血细胞的形态结构特点。

8.相关超微结构和功能可通过课堂讨论等完成。

Chapter 5　Blood

 Basic requirements for the experiment

1. Know the application of oil immersion lens.

2. Know the histological structures of bone marrow.

3. Familiar with the components of the blood and classifications of formed elements of the blood.

4. Master the size, morphology, structures and functions of erythrocyte. The normal range of erythrocyte, hemoglobin and reticulocyte.

5. Master the normal range and classifications of leukocyte. The normal range, shape, LM and EM structures and functions of different kinds of leukocyte.

6. Master the normal range, morphology, structures and functions of platelet.

7. Identify erythrocyte, neutrophilic granulocyte, eosinophilic granulocyte, basophilic granulocyte, monocyte, lymphocyte and platelet under LM.

8. The corresponding EM structures and functions will be discussed in lab.

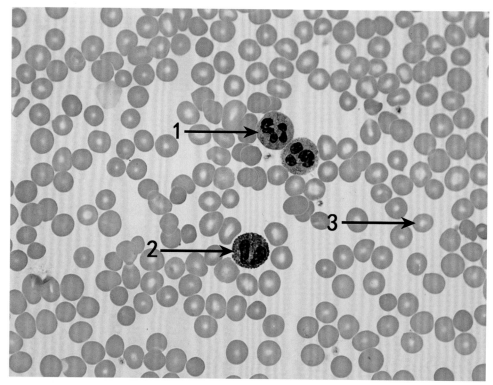

1. 中性粒细胞(neutrophilic granulocyte) 2. 嗜酸性粒细胞(eosinophilic granulocyte) 3. 红细胞(erythrocyte)

图 5-1 血涂片:人(Wright 染色,×100)

Pic. 5-1 Blood smear:Human. Wright staining ×100

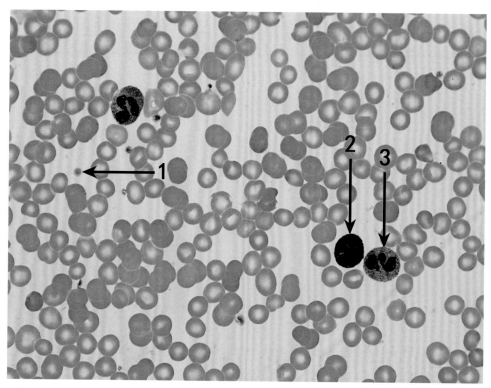

1. 血小板(platelet) 2. 嗜碱性粒细胞(basophilic granulocyte) 3. 中性粒细胞(neutrophilic granulocyte)

图 5-2 血涂片:人(Wright 染色,×100)

Pic. 5-2 Blood smear:Human. Wright staining ×100

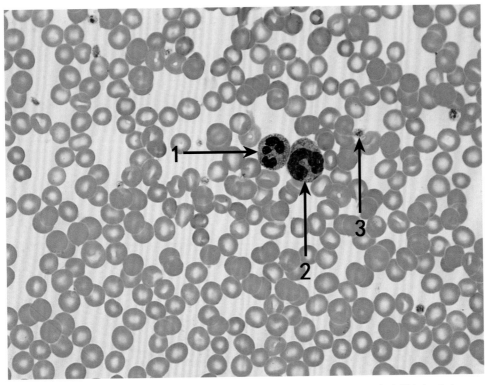

1. 中性粒细胞(neutrophilic granulocyte) 2. 单核细胞(monocyte) 3. 血小板(platelet)

图 5 - 3 血涂片:人(Wright 染色,×100)

Pic. 5 - 3 Blood smear:Human. Wright staining ×100

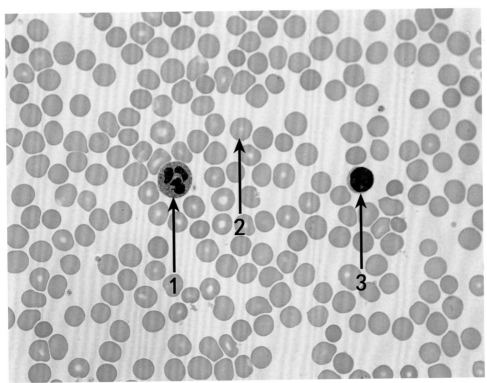

1. 中性粒细胞(neutrophilic granulocyte) 2. 红细胞(erythrocyte) 3. 淋巴细胞(lymphocyte)

图 5 - 4 血涂片:人(Wright 染色,×100)

Pic. 5 - 4 Blood smear:Human. Wright staining ×100

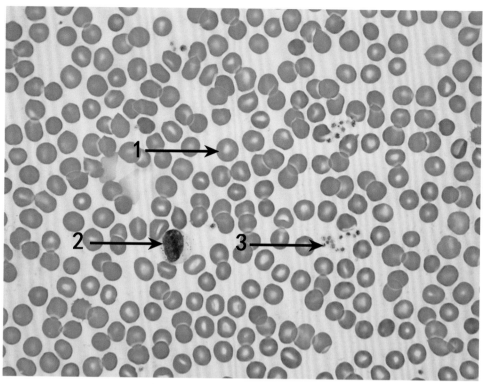

1.红细胞(erythrocyte) 2.淋巴细胞(lymphocyte) 3.血小板(platelets)

图 5-5 血涂片:人(Wright 染色,×100)

Pic. 5-5 Blood smear:Human. Wright staining ×100

第六章 肌组织

实验基本要求：

1. 了解骨骼肌的组织学结构。
2. 熟悉肌组织的一般结构特点和分类。
3. 掌握骨骼肌纤维、心肌纤维和平滑肌纤维的 LM 和 EM 结构特点。
4. 光镜下识别三种肌组织的形态结构特点。
5. 相关超微结构和功能可通过课堂讨论等完成。

Chapter 6　Muscle tissue

 Basic requirements for the experiment

1. Know the histological structures of skeletal muscle.
2. Familiar with the general structural features and classifications of the muscular tissue.
3. Master the LM and EM structural characteristics of skeletal muscle fiber, cardiac muscle fiber and smooth muscle fiber.
4. Identify skeletal muscle fiber, cardiac muscle fiber and smooth muscle fiber under LM.
5. The corresponding EM structures and functions will be discussed in lab.

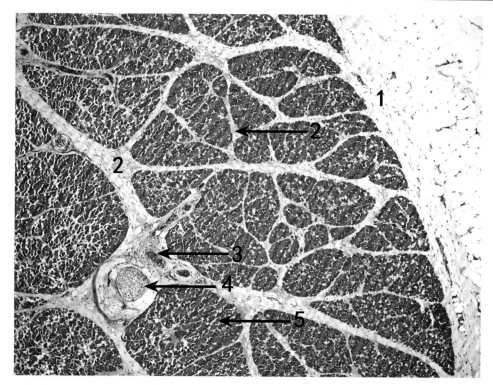

1.肌外膜（epimysium） 2.肌束膜（perimysium） 3.血管（blood vessel） 4.神经束（nerve bundle）
5.骨骼肌纤维横断面（cross section of skeletal muscle fiber）

图 6-1 骨骼肌：猫喉（HE 染色，×10）

Pic. 6-1 Skeletal muscle：Cat larynx. HE staining ×10

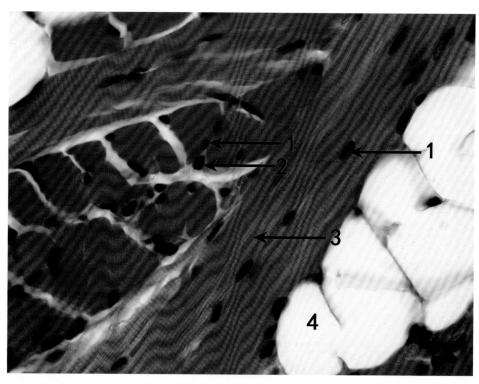

1.骨骼肌纤维的细胞核（nucleus of a skeletal muscle fiber） 2.肌内膜中成纤维细胞的细胞核（nucleus of a fibroblast in endomysium） 3.骨骼肌纤维纵断面示横纹（longitudinal section of a skeletal muscle fiber showing cross striation） 4.脂肪细胞（adipocyte）

图 6-2 骨骼肌纤维：猫舌（HE 染色，×100）

Pic. 6-2 Skeletal muscle fibers：Cat tongue. HE staining ×100

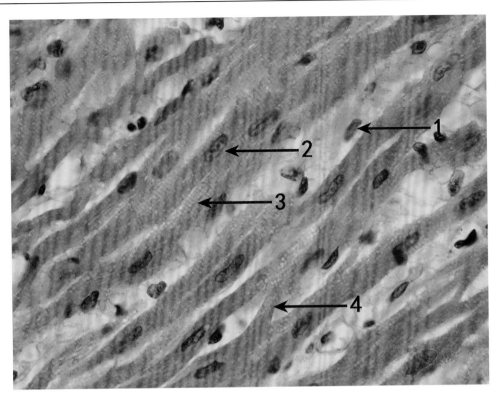

1. 成纤维细胞的细胞核(nucleus of a fibroblast) 2. 心肌纤维的细胞核(nucleus of a cardiac muscle fiber)

3. 心肌纤维纵断面示横纹(longitudinal section of a cardiac muscle fiber showing cross striation) 4. 心肌纤维分支(branch of a cardiac muscle fiber)

图 6 – 3 心肌纤维纵断:羊心脏(HE 染色,×100)

Pic. 6 – 3 Longitudinal section of cardiac muscle fibers:Sheep heart. HE staining ×100

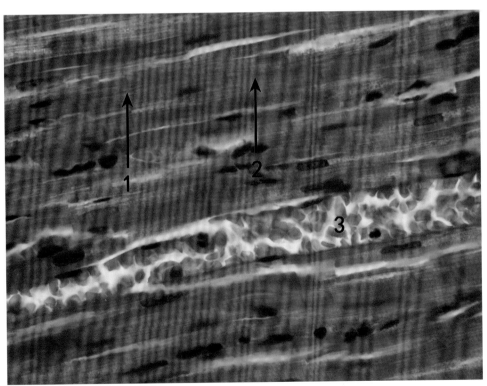

1. 闰盘(intercalated disk) 2. 横纹(cross striation) 3. 小血管(small blood vessel)

图 6 – 4 心肌闰盘:羊心脏(铁苏木素–伊红染色,×100)

Pic. 6 – 4 Intercalated disk of cardiac muscle:Sheep heart. Iron-hematoxylin Eosin staining ×100

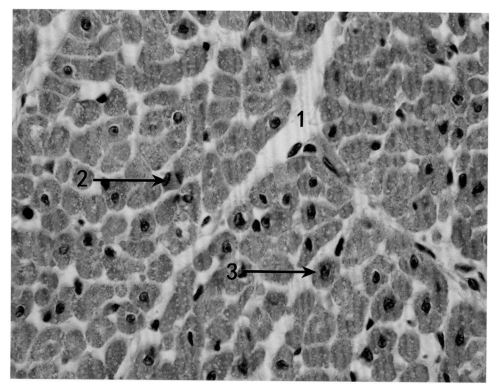

1.成束心肌纤维间的结缔组织(connective tissue among bundles of cardiac muscle fiber)

2.毛细血管(capillary) 3.心肌纤维的细胞核(nucleus of a cardiac muscle fiber)

图 6-5 心肌纤维横断:羊心脏(HE 染色,×100)

Pic. 6-5 Cross section of cardiac muscle fibers:Sheep heart. HE staining ×100

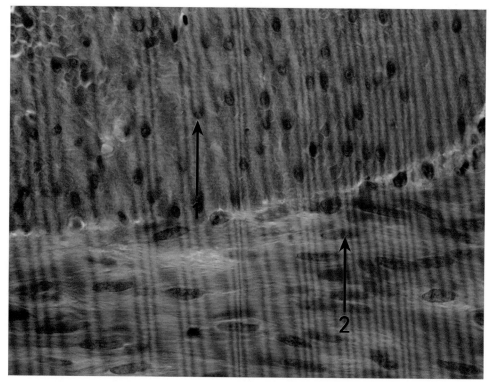

1.横断面上平滑肌纤维的细胞核(nucleus of a cross-sectioned smooth muscle fiber)

2.纵断面上平滑肌纤维的细胞核(nucleus of a longitudinally-sectioned smooth muscle fiber)

图 6-6 平滑肌纤维:猫空肠肠壁(HE 染色,×100)

Pic. 6-6 Smooth muscle fiber:Cat jejunal wall. HE staining ×100

第七章　神经组织

实验基本要求：

1. 了解神经的组织学结构。

2. 了解神经末梢的分类、结构和功能。

3. 熟悉神经纤维的分类和结构。掌握髓鞘的结构、功能和形成过程。

4. 掌握神经组织的组成和功能。

5. 掌握神经元胞体、轴突和树突的 LM 和 EM 结构和功能。

6. 掌握中枢和周围神经系统内神经胶质细胞的类型、形态特点和功能。

7. 光镜下识别神经元和有髓神经纤维。

8. 相关超微结构和功能可通过课堂讨论等完成。

Chapter 7　Nerve tissue

 Basic requirements for the experiment

1. Know the histological structures of nerve.

2. Know the classifications, structures and functions of nerve ending.

3. Familiar with the classifications and structures of nerve fiber. Master the structures, functions and formation processes of myelinated nerve fiber.

4. Master the structures and functions of nerve tissue.

5. Master the LM and EM structures and functions of neuron body, axon and dentrite.

6. Master the classifications, morphology and functions of neuroglial cell in central and periphery nervous system.

7. Identify neurons and myelinated nerve fiber under LM.

8. The corresponding EM structures and functions will be discussed in lab.

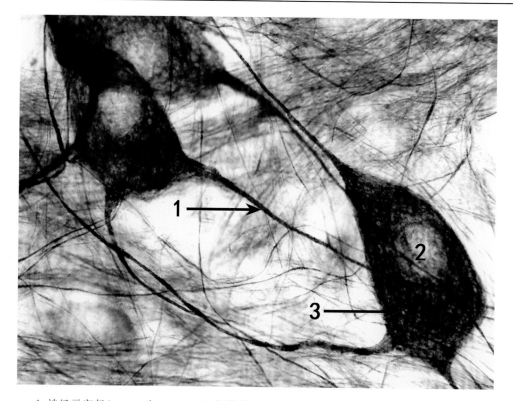

1.神经元突起(neuronal process) 2.细胞核(nucleus) 3.神经元胞体(neuronal cell body)

图 7－1　肠壁神经丛：猫(铺片,银染,×100)

Pic. 7－1　Nerve plexus of intestinal wall：Cat. Stretched preparation. Silver staining ×100

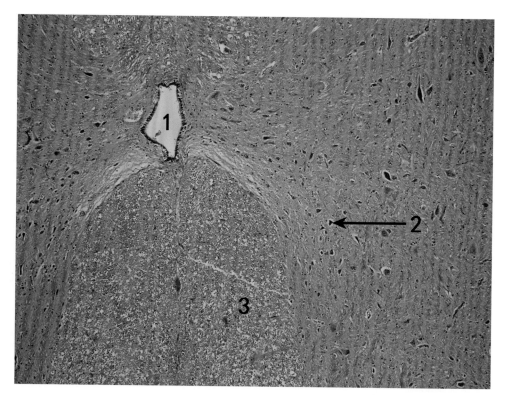

1.中央管(central canal) 2.灰质神经元(neuron in gray matter) 3.白质(white matter)

图 7－2　脊髓：猫(HE 染色,×10)

Pic. 7－2　Spinal cord：Cat. HE staining ×10

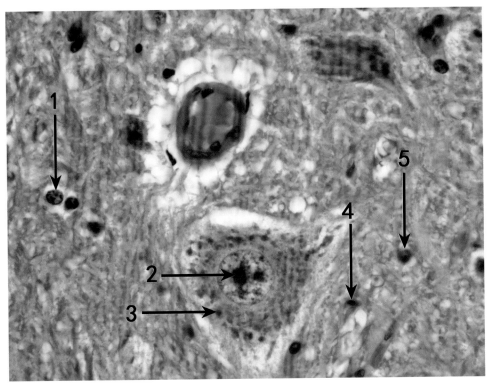

1.星形胶质细胞(astrocyte)　2.神经元核仁(nucleolus of a neuron)　3.尼氏体(Nissl body)

4.小胶质细胞(microglia)　5.少突胶质细胞(oligodendrocyte)

图 7-3　脊髓:猫(HE 染色,×100)

Pic. 7-3　Spinal cord:Cat. HE staining　×100

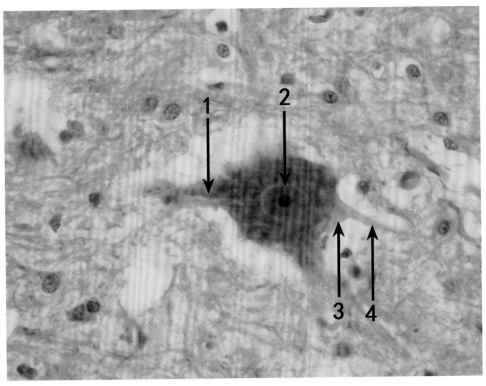

1.树突(dendrite)　2.神经元细胞核(nucleus of a neuron)　3.轴丘(axon hillock)　4.轴突(axon)

图 7-4　神经元:猫脊髓(HE 染色,×100)

Pic.7-4　Neuron:Cat spinal cord. HE staining　×100

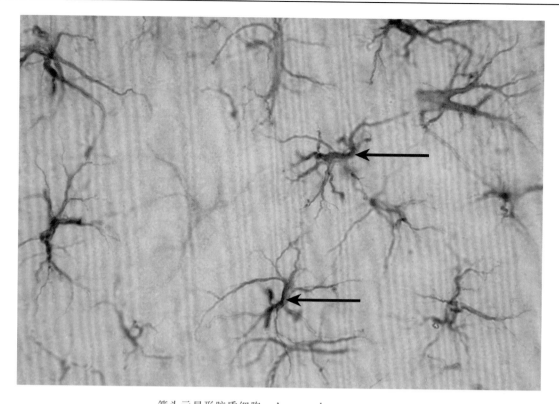

箭头示星形胶质细胞。Arrows show astrocytes.

图 7 - 5　星形胶质细胞:小鼠大脑皮质(GFAP 免疫酶染色,DAB 显色,×100)

Pic. 7 - 5　Astrocyte:Brain cortex of mouse cerebrum. GFAP immunoenzyme staining,DAB visualization　×100

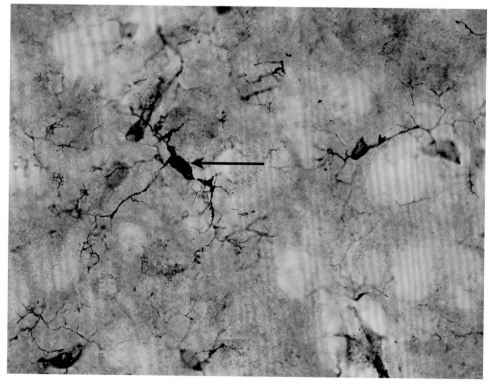

箭头示少突胶质细胞。The arrow shows an oligodendrocyte.

图 7 - 6　少突胶质细胞:猫小脑(银染,×100)

Pic. 7 - 6　Oligodendrocyte:Cat cerebellum. Silver staining　×100

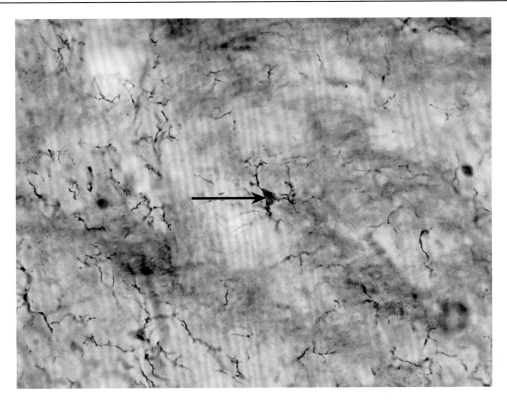

箭头示小胶质细胞。The arrow shows a microglial cell.

图 7 - 7 小胶质细胞(猫小脑(银染,×100)

Pic. 7 - 7 Microglia:Cat cerebella. Silver staining ×100

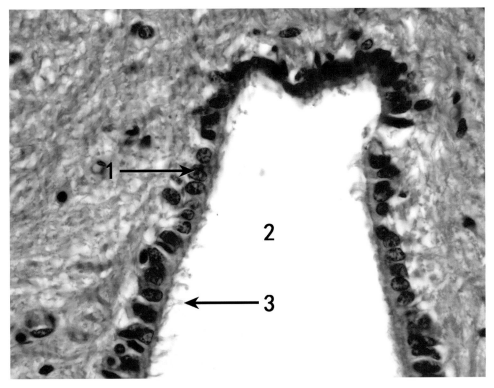

1.室管膜细胞(ependymal cell) 2.中央管(central canal) 3.纤毛(cilia of ependymal cell)

图 7 - 8 室管膜细胞:猫脊髓(HE 染色,×100)

Pic. 7 - 8 Ependymal cells:Cat spinal cord. HE staining ×100

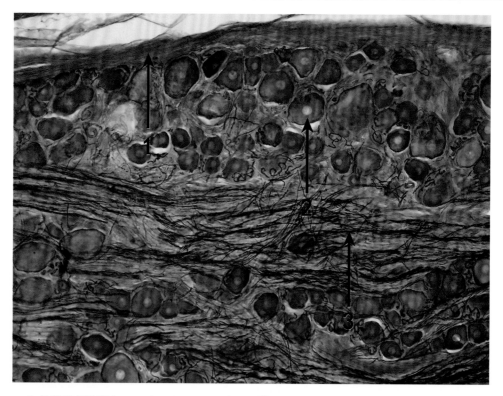

1. 结缔组织被膜（connective tissue capsule） 2. 神经元（neuron） 3. 神经纤维（nerve fibers）

图 7 - 9 脊神经节：人（银染，×20）。

Pic. 7 - 9 Spinal ganglion：Human. Silver staining ×20

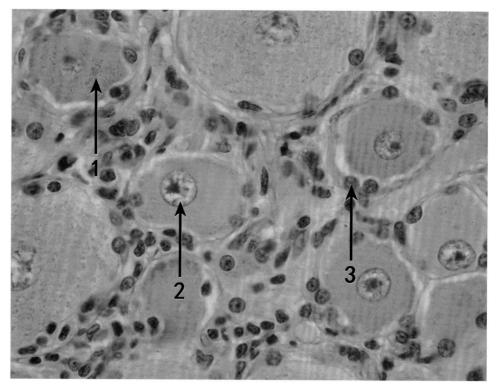

1. 脂褐素（lipofuscin） 2. 神经元细胞核（nucleus of a neuron） 3. 卫星细胞（satellite cell）

图 7 - 10 脊神经节：人（HE 染色，×100）

Pic. 7 - 10 Spinal ganglion：Human. HE staining ×100

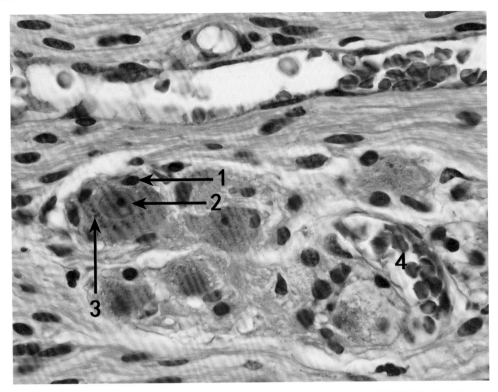

1.卫星细胞（satellite cell）　2.神经元细胞核（nucleus of a neuron）　3.脂褐素（lipofuscin）

4.小血管（small blood vessel）

图 7 - 11　交感神经节：人（HE 染色，×100）

Pic. 7 - 11　Sympathetic ganglion：Human.　HE staining　×100

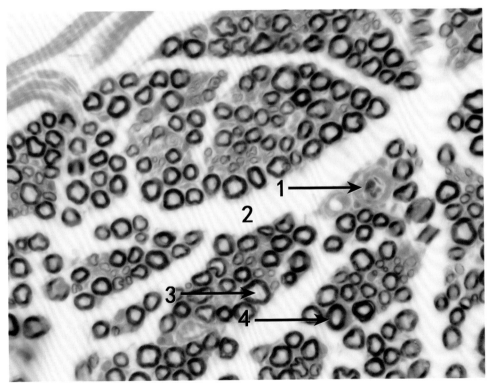

1.毛细血管（capillary）　2.神经束膜（perineurium）　3.轴突（axon）　4.髓鞘（myelin sheath）

图 7 - 12　坐骨神经横断面：猫（四氧化锇染色，×100）

Pic. 7 - 12　Cross section of sciatic nerve：Cat.　Osmium tetroxide staining　×100

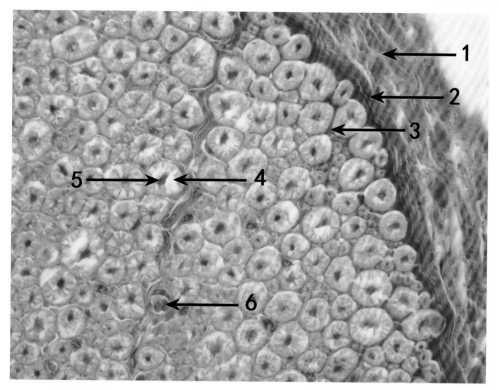

1.神经外膜(epineurium) 2.神经束膜(perineurium) 3.神经内膜(endoneurium)
4.髓鞘(myelin sheath) 5.轴突(axon) 6.毛细血管(capillary)
图 7-13 坐骨神经横断面:猫(HE 染色,×100)
Pic. 7-13 Cross section of sciatic nerve:Cat. HE staining ×100

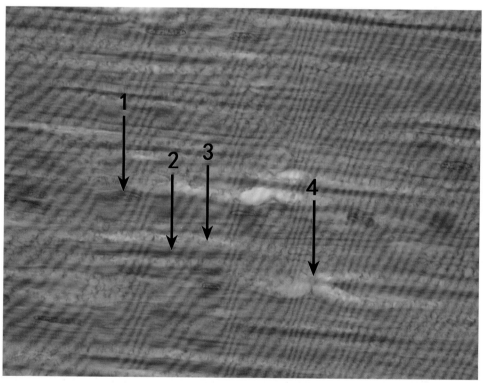

1.施万细胞胞核(nucleus of a Schwann cell) 2.轴突(axon) 3.髓鞘(myelin sheath) 4.郎飞结(Ranvier node)
图 7-14 坐骨神经纵断面:猫(HE 染色,×100)
Pic. 7-14 Longitudinal section of sciatic nerve:Cat. HE staining ×100

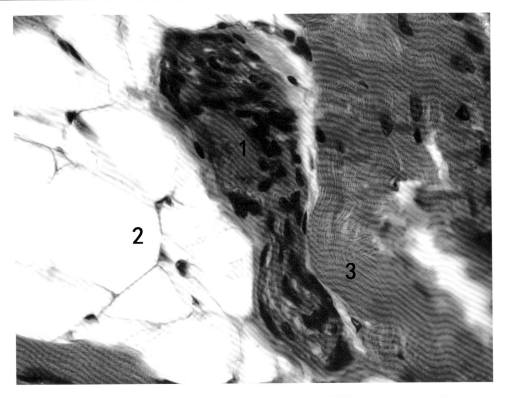

1.神经斑(nerve plaque)　2.脂肪细胞(fat cell)　3.骨骼肌纤维(skeletal muscle fiber)

图 7 - 15　神经斑:猫舌(HE 染色,×100)

Pic. 7 - 15　Nerve plaque:Cat tongue. HE staining　×100

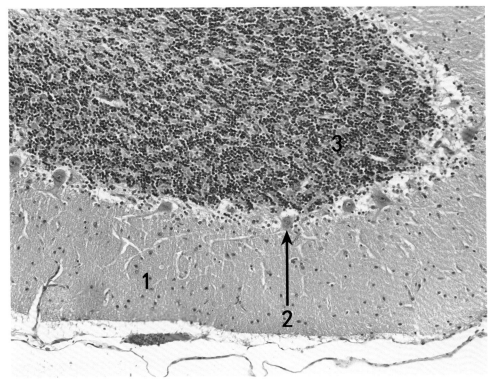

1.分子层(molecular layer)　2.浦肯野细胞层(Purkinje cell layer)　3.颗粒层(granular layer)

图 7 - 16　小脑皮质:猫(HE 染色,×20)

Pic. 7 - 16　Cerebellar cortex:Cat. HE staining　×20

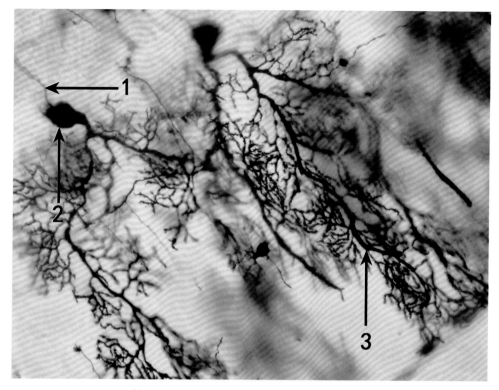

1.轴突（axon） 2.胞体（cell body） 3.树突（dendrite）

图 7-17 浦肯野细胞：猫小脑皮质（银染，×100）

Pic. 7-17 Purkinje cell：Cat cerebellar cortex. Silver staining ×100

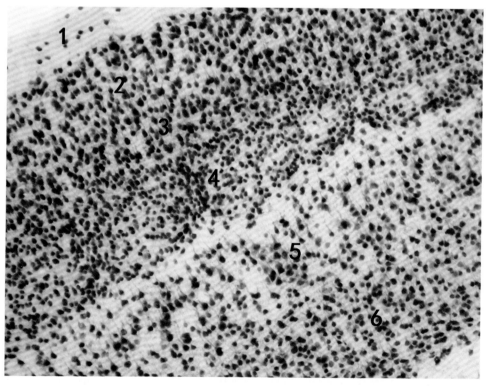

1.分子层（molecular layer） 2.外颗粒层（external granular layer） 3.外锥体细胞层（external pyramidal layer）

4.内颗粒层（internal granular layer） 5.内锥体细胞层（internal pyramidal layer） 6.多形细胞层等（polymorphic layer）

图 7-18 大脑新皮质：小鼠（NEUN 免疫酶染色，DAB 显色，×20）

Pic. 7-18 Cerebral neocortex：Cat. NEUN immunoenzyme staining，DAB visualization ×20

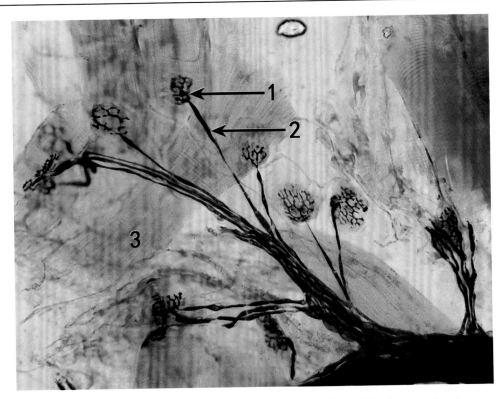

1.运动终板(motor end plate) 2.轴突(axon) 3.骨骼肌纤维(skeletal muscle fiber)

图 7-19 运动终板:兔肋间肌(压片,氯化金染色,×40)

Pic. 7-19 Motor end plate:Rabbit intercostal muscle. Tabletting. Gold chloride staining ×40

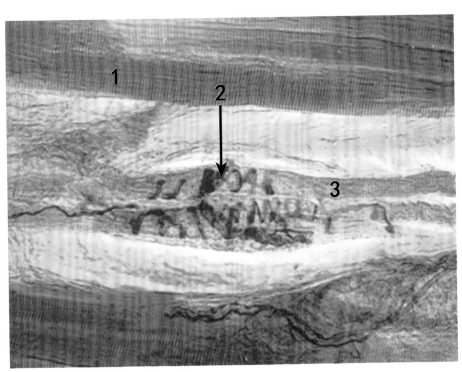

1.梭外肌(extrafusal muscle fiber) 2.缠绕梭内肌的神经纤维(nerve fiber) 3.梭内肌(intrafusal muscle fiber)

图 7-20 肌梭:猫骨骼肌(银染,×40)

Pic. 7-20 Muscle spindle:Cat skeletal muscle. Silver staining ×40

第八章　循环系统

实验基本要求：

1. 熟悉血管壁的一般组织结构。
2. 熟悉中动脉、大动脉、小动脉、微动脉和静脉的组织结构和功能。
3. 掌握三类毛细血管分类、分布、LM 和 EM 结构及功能。
4. 掌握心壁的组织学结构和功能。
5. 光镜下识别心脏壁、中动静脉、大动脉、小动脉、静脉和毛细血管。
6. 相关超微结构和功能可通过课堂讨论等完成。

Chapter 8　Circulatory system

 Basic requirements for the experiment

1. Familiar with the general structures of blood vessel wall.

2. Familiar with the histological structures and functions of medium-sized, large and small artery, arteriole and veins.

3. Master the classifications, distributions, LM and EM structures and functions of three types of capillaries.

4. Master the histological structures and functions of heart wall.

5. Identify heart wall, medium-sized arteries and veins, large and small artery, vein and capillary under LM.

6. The corresponding EM structures and functions will be discussed in lab.

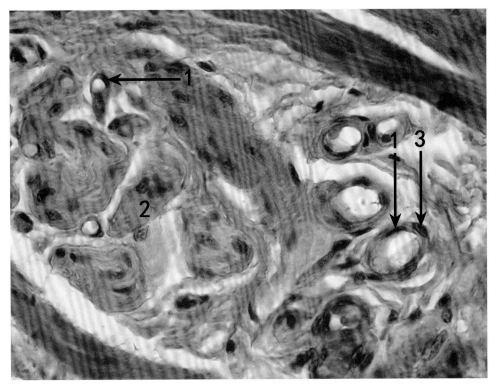

1.毛细血管内皮细胞（endothelial cell of capillary）　2.肌间神经丛（myenteric nervous plexus）　3.周细胞（pericyte）

图 8 - 1　毛细血管:猫胃底（HE 染色,×100）

Pic. 8 - 1　Capillary:Cat gastric fundus. HE staining　×100

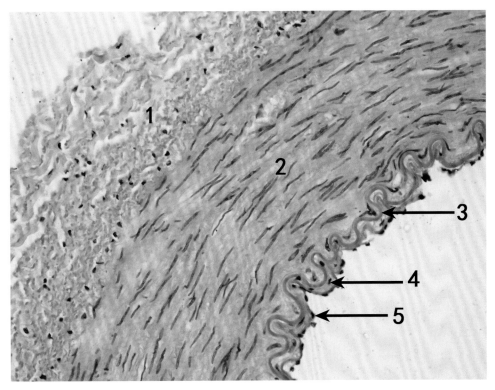

1.外膜（tunica adventitia）　2.中膜（tunica media）　3.内弹性膜（internal elastic membrane）

4.内皮下层（subendothelial layer）　5.内皮（endothelium）

图 8 - 2　中动脉:兔（HE 染色,×40）

Pic. 8 - 2　Medium-sized artery:Rabbit. HE staining　×40

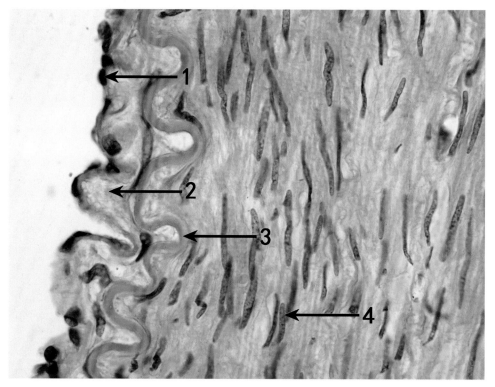

1. 内皮（endothelium） 2. 内皮下层（subendothelial layer） 3. 内弹性膜（internal elastic membrane）
4. 中膜平滑肌（smooth muscle in tunica media）

图 8-3　中动脉：兔（HE 染色，×100）

Pic. 8-3　Medium-sized artery：Rabbit. HE staining　×100

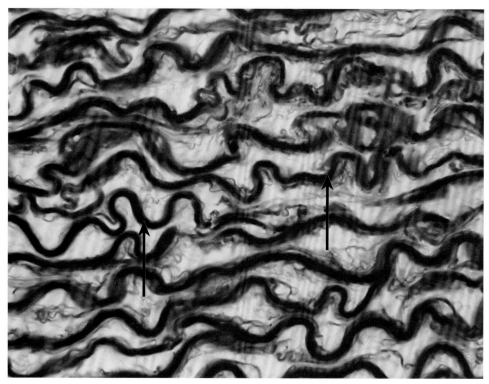

箭头示弹性膜。Arrows show elastic membranes.

图 8-4　大动脉中膜：人（醛复红染色，×100）

Pic. 8-4　Tunica media of large artery：Human. Aldehyde-fuchsin staining　×100

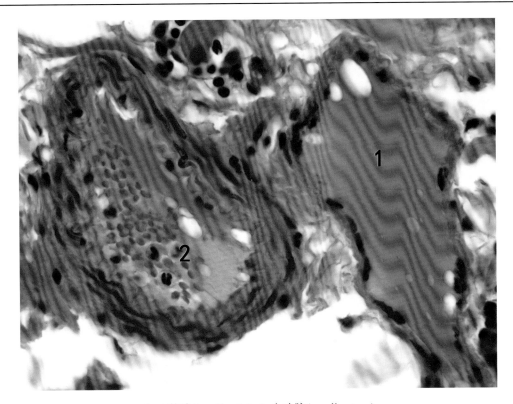

1.小静脉(small vein)　2.小动脉(small artery)

图 8-5　小动脉和小静脉:猫小肠(HE 染色,×100)

Pic. 8-5　Small artery and small vein:Cat small intestine.　HE staining　×100

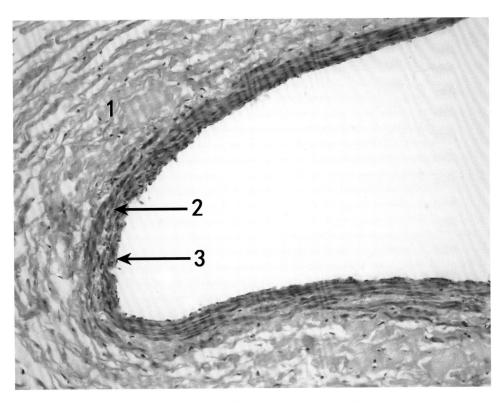

1.外膜(tunica adventitia)　2.中膜(tunica media)　3.内膜(tunica intima)

图 8-6　中静脉:兔(HE 染色,×20)

Pic. 8-6　Medium-sized vein:Rabbit.　HE staining　×20

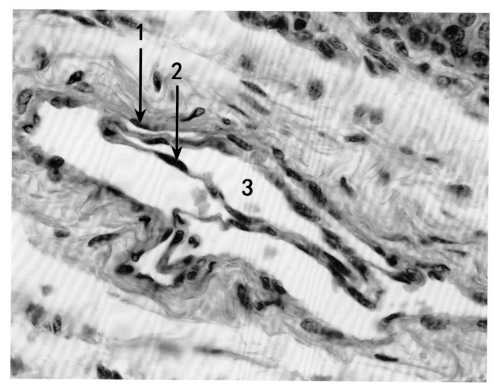

1. 静脉内皮（endothelium of vein） 2. 静脉瓣（venous valve） 3. 静脉管腔（venous lumen）

图 8 - 7　静脉瓣：兔（HE 染色，×100）

Pic. 8 - 7　Vein valve：Rabbit. HE staining　×100

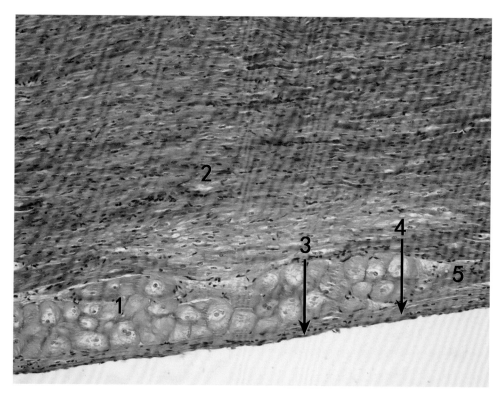

1. 浦肯野纤维（Purkinje fibers） 2. 心肌膜（myocardium） 3. 内皮（endothelium）

4. 内皮下层（subendothelial layer） 5. 心内膜下层（subendocardial layer）

图 8 - 8　心脏：羊（HE 染色，×20）

Pic. 8 - 8　Heart：Sheep. HE staining　×20

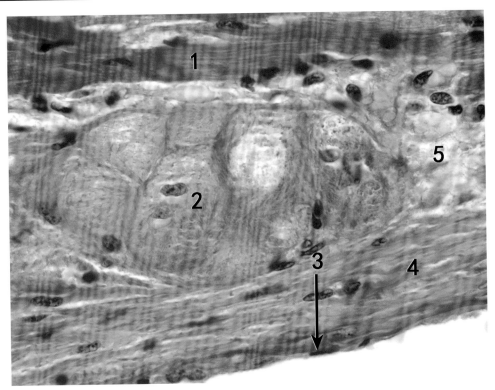

1.普通心肌纤维（ordinary cardiac muscle cell）　2.浦肯野纤维（Purkinje fiber）　3.内皮（endothelium）
4.内皮下层（subendothelial layer）　5.心内膜下层（subendocardial layer）

图 8 - 9　心内膜：羊（HE 染色，×100）

Pic. 8 - 9　Endocardium：Sheep. HE staining　×100

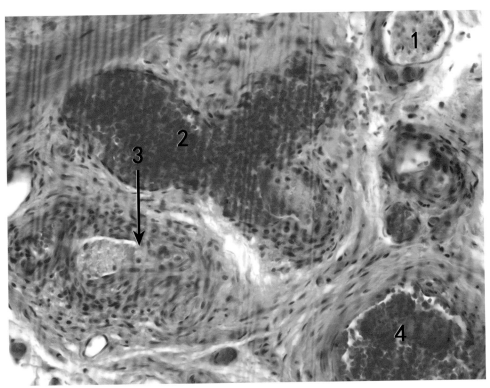

1.神经束（nerve bundle）　2.微静脉（venule）　3.动静脉吻合（arteriovenous anastomosis）　4.小静脉（small artery）

图 8 - 10　动静脉吻合：人指皮真皮（HE 染色，×100）

Pic. 8 - 10　Arteriovenous anastomosis：Dermis of human finger skin. HE staining　×100

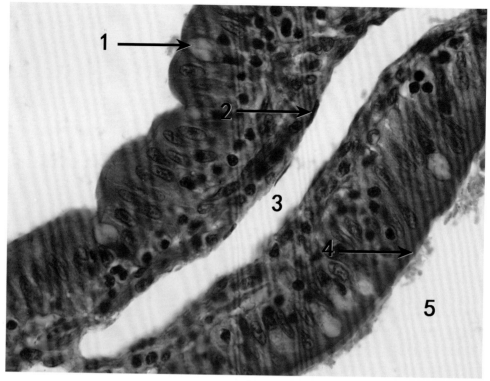

1.杯状细胞(goblet cell) 2.内皮(endothelium) 3.淋巴管/中央乳糜管(lymphatic vessel/central lacteal)

4.纹状缘(striated border) 5.肠腔(jejunum lumen)

图8-11 淋巴管:猫空肠(HE染色,×100)

Pic. 8-11 Lymphatic vessel:Cat jejunum. HE staining ×100

第九章 免疫系统

实验基本要求：

1. 了解免疫系统的组成与功能。

2. 了解扁桃体的组织结构和功能。

3. 熟悉淋巴组织的结构、类型和分布。

4. 熟悉胸腺的组织结构：胸腺皮质、髓质和胸腺小体的结构。

5. 掌握淋巴结的组织结构：被膜、小梁、被膜下窦、小梁周窦、皮质、淋巴小结、副皮质区、髓质、髓窦、髓索。

6. 掌握脾的组织结构：被膜、小梁、白髓、动脉周围淋巴鞘、脾小体、边缘区、红髓、脾索和脾窦。

7. 光镜下识别胸腺、淋巴结和脾。

8. 相关超微结构和功能可通过课堂讨论等完成。

Chapter 9　Immune system

 Basic requirements for the experiment

1. Know the compositions and functions of immune system.

2. Know the histological structures and function of tonsil.

3. Familiar with the histological, classifications structures and functions of lymphatic tissue.

4. Familiar with the histological structures of thymus：cortex，medulla and thymic corpuscle.

5. Master the histological structures of lymph node：capsule，subcapsular sinus，trabecula，peritrabecular sinus，cortex，lymphoid nodule，paracortical zone，medulla，lymphatic sinus and medullary cord.

6. Master the histological structures of spleen：capsule，trabecula，white pulp，periarterial lymphatic sheath，splenic corpuscle，marginal zone，red pulp，splenic cord and splenic sinusoid.

7. Identify thymus，lymph node and spleen under LM.

8. The corresponding EM structures and functions will be discussed in lab.

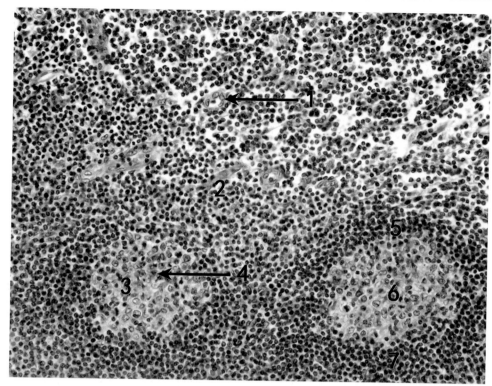

1.毛细血管后微静脉(postcapillary venule) 2.弥散淋巴组织(diffuse lymphoid tissue) 3.淋巴小结(lymphoid nodule)
4.生发中心(germinal center) 5.暗区(dark zone) 6.明区(light zone) 7.小结帽(nodule cap)

图9-1 淋巴组织:狗淋巴结(HE染色,×40)

Pic. 9-1 Lymphaoid tissue:Dog lymph node. HE staining ×40

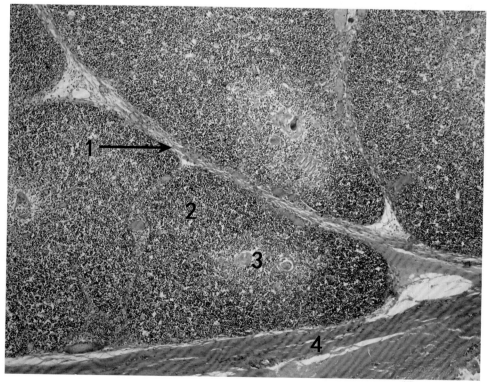

1.小叶间隔(interlobular septum) 2.皮质(cortex) 3.髓质(medulla) 4.被膜(capsule)

图9-2 胸腺:人胎儿(HE染色,×10)

Pic. 9-2 Thymus:Human fetus. HE staining ×10

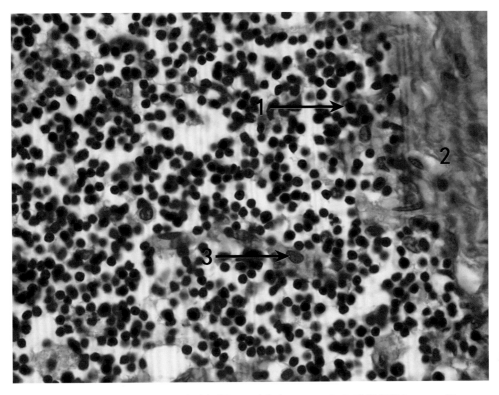

1.胸腺细胞(thymocyte) 2.小叶间隔(interlobular septum) 3.哺育细胞(nurse cell)

图 9-3 胸腺皮质：人胎儿(HE 染色，×100)

Pic. 9-3 Thymic cortex：Human fetus. HE staining ×100

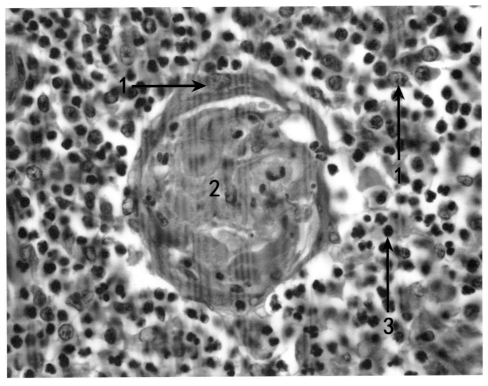

1.胸腺上皮细胞(thymic epithelial cell) 2.胸腺小体(thymic corpuscle) 3.胸腺细胞(thymocyte)

图 9-4 胸腺小体：人胎儿(HE 染色，×100)

Pic. 9-4 Thymic corpuscle：Human fetus. HE staining ×100

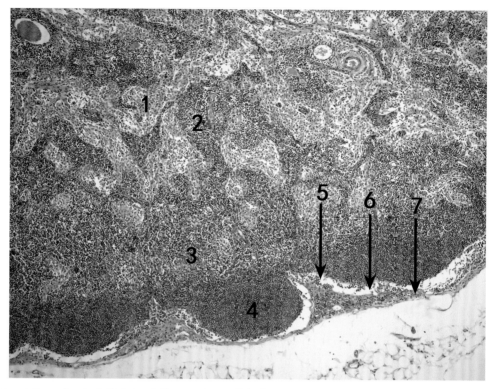

1.髓窦（medullary sinus） 2.髓索（medullary cord） 3.副皮质区（paracortical zone） 4.淋巴小结（lymphoid nodule）
5.小梁周窦（peritrabecular sinus） 6.被膜下窦（subcapsular sinus） 7.被膜（capsule）

图 9-5 淋巴结：狗（HE 染色，×20）

Pic. 9-5 Lymph node：Dog. HE staining ×20

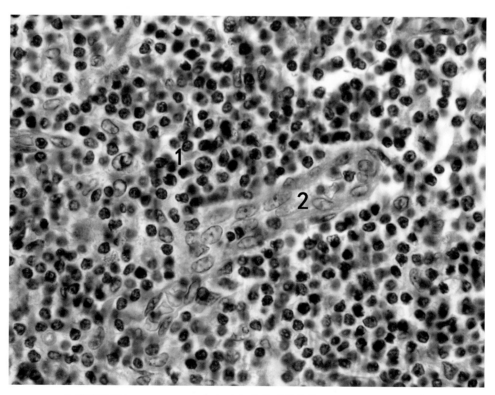

1.副皮质区（paracortex zone） 2.毛细血管后微静脉（postcapillary venule）

图 9-6 淋巴结副皮质区：狗（HE 染色，×100）

Pic. 9-6 Paracortex zone of lymph node：Dog. HE staining ×100

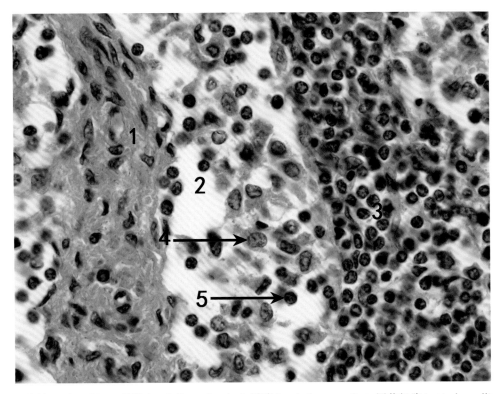

1. 小梁（trabecula）　2. 髓窦（medullary sinus）　3. 髓索（medullary cord）　4. 网状细胞（reticular cell）

5. 淋巴细胞（lymphocyte）

图 9 - 7　淋巴结髓质：狗（HE 染色，×100）

Pic. 9 - 7　Medulla of lymph node：Dog. HE staining　×100

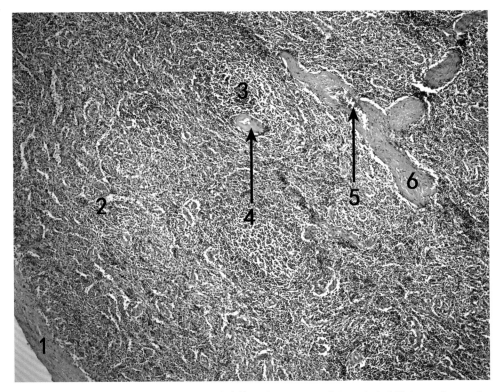

1. 被膜（capsule）　2. 红髓（red pulp）　3. 脾小体（splenic corpuscle）　4. 中央动脉（central artery）

5. 小梁静脉（trabecular vein）　6. 小梁（trabecula）

图 9 - 8　脾：猫（HE 染色，×20）

Pic. 9 - 8　Spleen：Cat. HE staining　×20

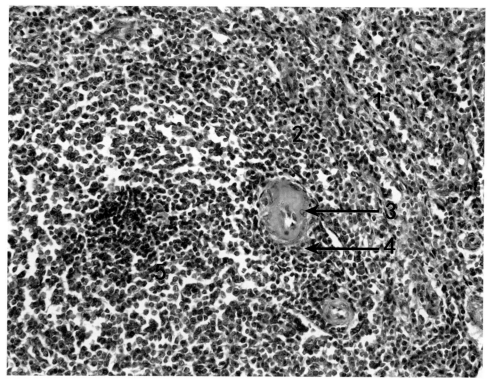

1.红髓(red pulp) 2.边缘区(marginal zone) 3.中央动脉(central artery)

4.动脉周围淋巴鞘(periarterial lymphatic sheath) 5.脾小体(splenic corpuscle)

图9-9 脾白髓:猫(HE染色,×40)

Pic.9-9 White pulp of spleen:Cat. HE staining ×40

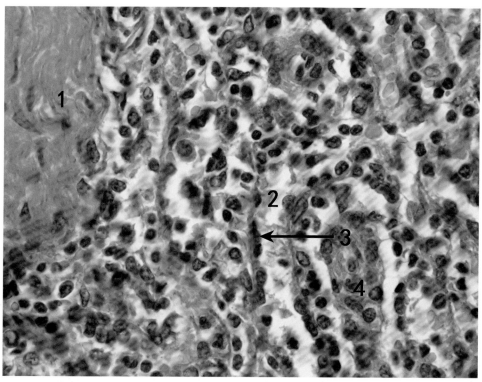

1.小梁(trabecula) 2.脾窦(splenic sinusoid) 3.脾窦内皮(endothelium of splenic sinusoid) 4.脾索(splenic cord)

图9-10 脾红髓:猫(HE染色,×100)

Pic.9-10 Red pulp of spleen:Cat. HE staining ×100

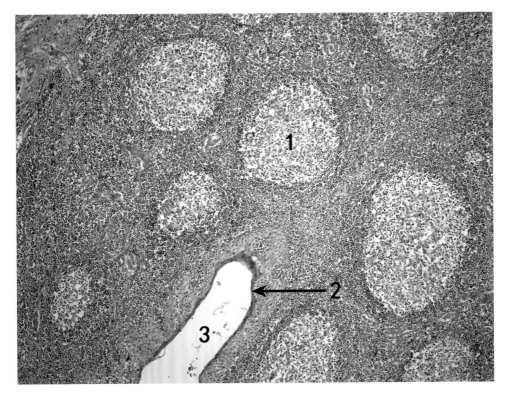

1.淋巴小结（lymphatic nodule） 2.隐窝上皮（crypt epithelium） 3.隐窝（crypt）

图 9－11 腭扁桃体：人（HE 染色，×4）

Pic. 9－11 Palatine tonsil：Human. HE staining ×4

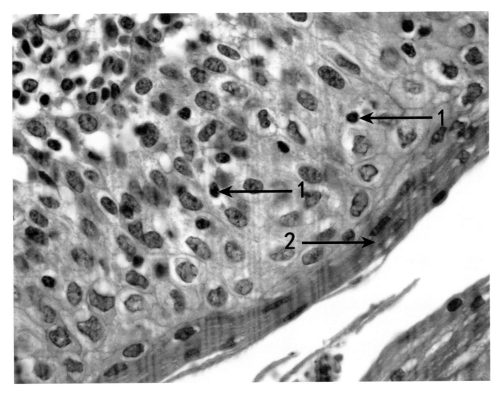

1.淋巴细胞（lymphocyte） 2.复层扁平上皮表层（superficial layer of stratified squamous epithelium）

图 9－12 淋巴上皮组织：人腭扁桃体（HE 染色，×100）

Pic. 9－12 Lymphoepithelial tissue：Human palatine tonsil. HE staining ×100

第十章 内分泌系统

实验基本要求：

1.了解垂体的分部。掌握腺垂体远侧部三种腺细胞以及神经部赫令体的结构特点及功能。

2.熟悉内分泌系统的组成。内分泌腺的共同结构特点以及两类内分泌细胞的 EM 结构特点。

3.熟悉甲状旁腺的结构特点与功能。

4.掌握肾上腺皮质球状带、束状带、网状带和髓质的 LM 和 EM 结构和功能。

5.掌握甲状腺的组织结构。滤泡上皮细胞、胶质、滤泡旁细胞的 LM 和 EM 结构和功能。

6.光镜下识别甲状腺、肾上腺和垂体。

7.相关超微结构和功能可通过课堂讨论等完成。

Chapter 10 Endocrine system

 Basic requirements for the experiment

1. Know the divisions of pituitary gland. Master the functions of three cell types in pars distalis of the adenohypophysis, structures and functions of Herring bodies in neurohypophysis.

2. Familiar with the compositions of endocrine system. The general structural features of the endocrine glands and EM structural characteristics of two types of endocrine cells.

3. Familiar with the structures and functions of parathyroid gland.

4. Master the LM and EM structures and functions of zona glomerulosa, zona fasciculata, zona reticularis and medulla of the adrenal gland.

5. Master the histological structures of thyroid. The LM and EM structures and functions of follicular epithelial cell, colloid and parafollicular cell.

6. Identify thyroid, adrenal gland and pituitary gland under LM.

7. The corresponding EM structures and functions will be discussed in lab.

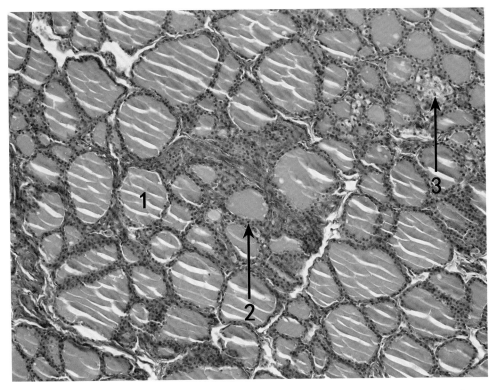

1. 滤泡胶质（colloid）　2. 滤泡上皮（follicular epithelium）　3. 滤泡旁细胞（parafollicular cells）

图 10 - 1　甲状腺：人（HE 染色，×20）

Pic. 10 - 1　Thyroid gland：Human. HE staining　×20

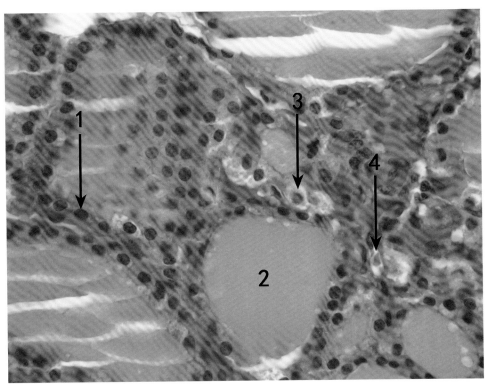

1. 滤泡上皮细胞（follicular epithelial cell）　2. 胶质（colloid）　3. 滤泡旁细胞（parafollicular cell）　4. 毛细血管（capillary）

图 10 - 2　甲状腺：人（HE 染色，×100）

Pic. 10 - 2　Thyroid gland：Human. HE staining　×100

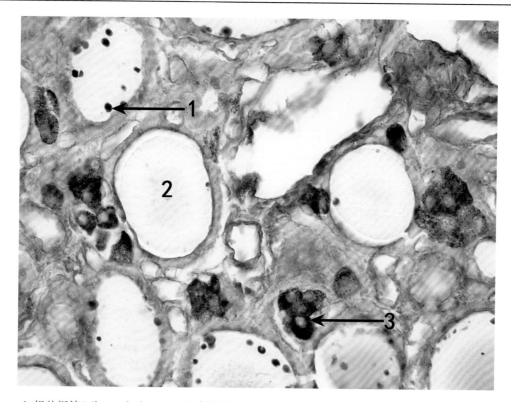

1. 银盐沉淀（silver salt deposit） 2. 滤泡腔（follicular cavity） 3. 滤泡旁细胞（parafollicular cell）

图 10－3　甲状腺：人（银染，×100）

Pic. 10－3　Thyroid gland：Human. Silver staining　×100

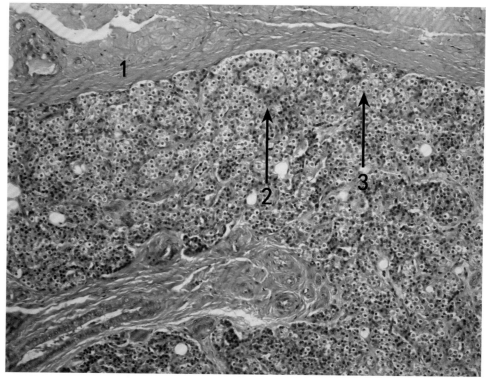

1. 被膜（capsule） 2. 嗜酸性细胞（oxyphil cell） 3. 主细胞（chief cell）

图 10－4　甲状旁腺：大鼠（HE 染色，×20）

Pic. 10－4　Parathyroid gland：Rat. HE staining　×20

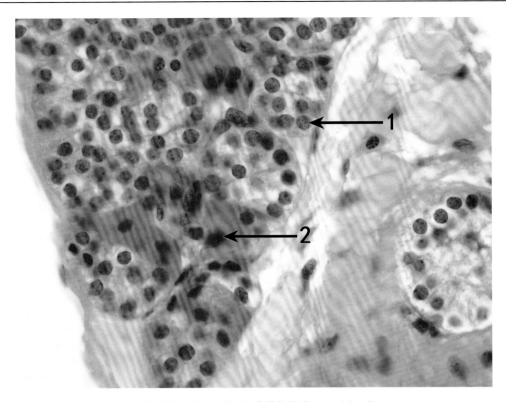

1. 主细胞(chief cell)　2. 嗜酸性细胞(oxyphil cell)

图 10 - 5　甲状旁腺：大鼠(HE 染色，×100)

Pic. 10 - 5　Parathyroid gland：Rat. HE staining　×100

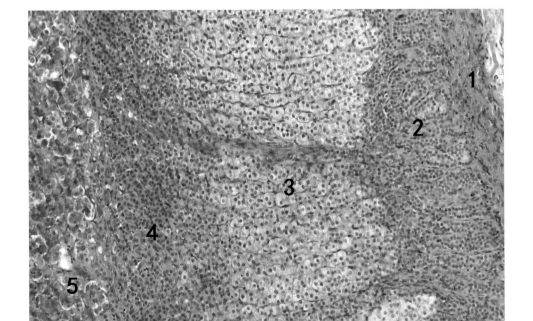

1. 被膜(capsule)　2. 球状带(zona glomerulosa)　3. 束状带(zona fasciculata)　4. 网状带(zona reticularis)　5. 髓质(medulla)

图 10 - 6　肾上腺：兔(HE 染色，×20)

Pic. 10 - 6　Adrenal gland：Rabbit. HE staining　×20

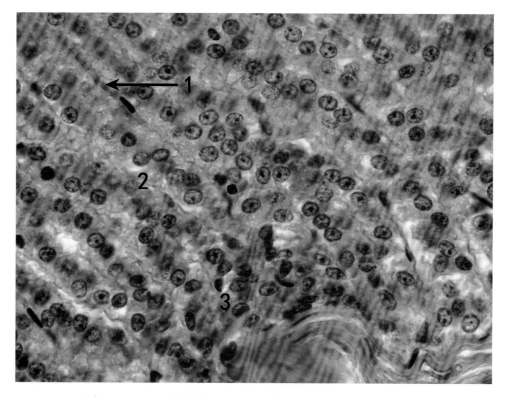

1.血窦(sinusoid) 2.束状带(zona fasciculata) 3.球状带(zona glomerulosa)

图 10 – 7　肾上腺：兔(HE 染色，×100)

Pic. 10 – 7　Adrenal gland：Rabbit. HE staining　×100

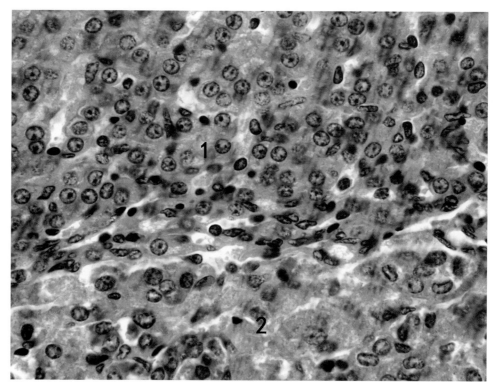

1.网状带(zona reticularis) 2.髓质(medulla)

图 10 – 8　肾上腺：兔(HE 染色，×100)

Pic. 10 – 8　Adrenal gland：Rabbit. HE staining　×100

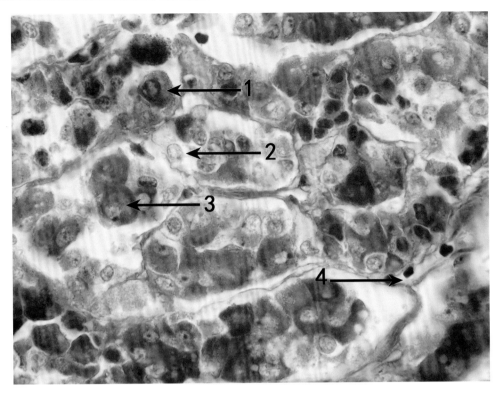

1. 嗜酸性细胞（acidophilic cell） 2. 嫌色细胞（chromophobe cell） 3. 嗜碱性细胞（basophilic cell） 4. 血窦（sinusoid）

图 10 - 9 垂体远侧部：猪（三色染色，×100）

Pic. 10 - 9 Pars distalis of hypophysis：Pig. Trichrome staining ×100

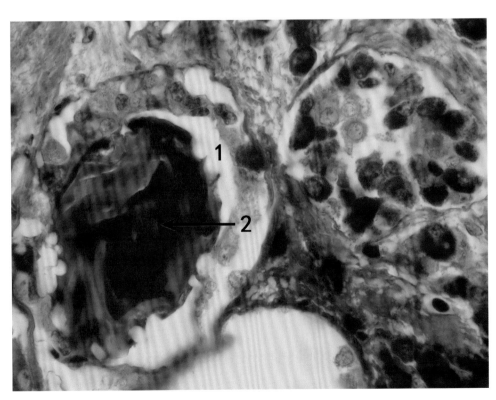

1. 滤泡（follicle） 2. 滤泡腔中的胶质（colloid in follicular cavity）

图 10 - 10 垂体中间部：猪（三色染色，×100）

Pic. 10 - 10 Pars intermedia of hypophysis：Pig. Trichrome staining ×100

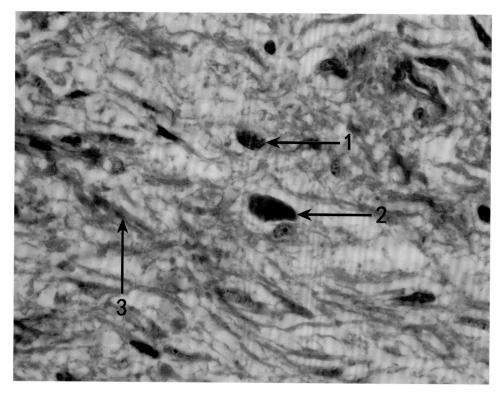

1.垂体细胞(pituicyte) 2.赫令体(Herring body) 3.无髓神经纤维(unmyelinated nerve fiber)

图 10 - 11　垂体神经部:猪(三色染色,×100)

Pic. 10 - 11　Pars nervosa of hypophysis:Pig. Trichrome staining　×100

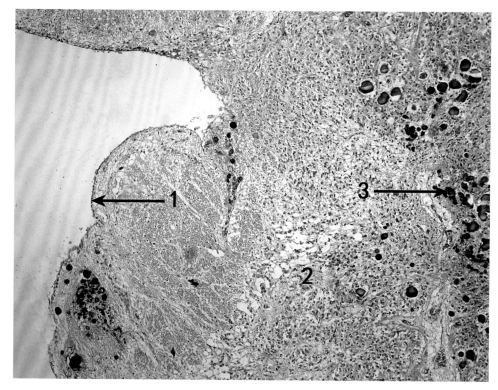

1.软脑膜(cerebral pia mater) 2.松果体实质(parenchyma of pineal body) 3.脑砂(brain sand)

图 10 - 12　松果体:人(HE 染色,×10)

Pic. 10 - 12　Pineal body:Human. HE staining　×10

第十一章 皮 肤

实验基本要求：

1. 了解真皮乳头层和网织层的结构。

2. 了解皮肤附属器的结构和功能：毛、皮脂腺、汗腺、指（趾）甲。

3. 熟悉皮肤的组成和功能。

4. 掌握表皮 5 层的组织学结构和功能。

5. 光镜下识别指皮和头皮。

6. 相关超微结构和功能可通过课堂讨论等完成。

Chapter 11　Skin

 Basic requirements for the experiment

1. Know the structure of papillary layer and reticular layer of dermis.

2. Know the structural and functions of skin appendage: hair, sebaceous gland, sweat gland and nail.

3. Familiar with the compositions and functions of skin.

4. Master the structures and functions of five layers of epidermis.

5. Identify finger skin and scalp under LM.

6. The corresponding EM structures and functions will be discussed in lab.

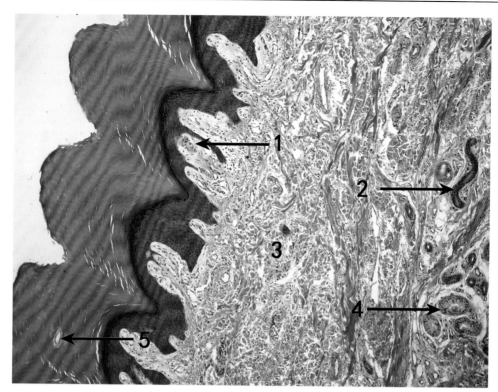

1. 真皮乳头层内的触觉小体 (tactile corpuscle in papillary layer of dermis) 2. 汗腺导管 (duct of sweat gland)

3. 真皮网织层 (reticular layer of dermis) 4. 汗腺分泌部 (secretory portion of sweat gland)

5. 表皮角化层内的汗腺导管 (duct of sweat gland in stratum corneum of epidermis)

图 11-1 皮肤：人指皮 (HE 染色，×10)

Pic. 11-1 Skin：Human finger skin. HE staining ×10

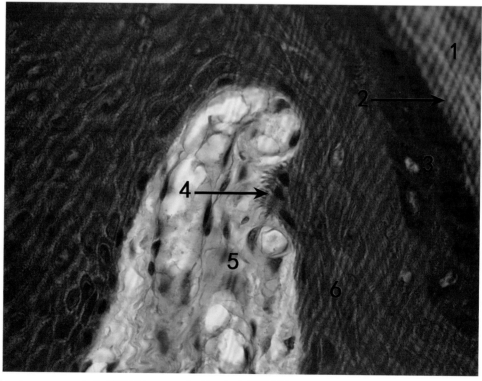

1. 角质层 (stratum corneum) 2. 透明层 (stratum lucidum) 3. 颗粒层 (stratum granulosum) 4. 基底层 (stratum basale)

5. 真皮乳头层 (papillary layer of dermis) 6. 棘层 (stratum spinosum)

图 11-2 表皮：人指皮 (HE 染色，×100)

Pic. 11-2 Epidermis：Human finger skin. HE staining ×100

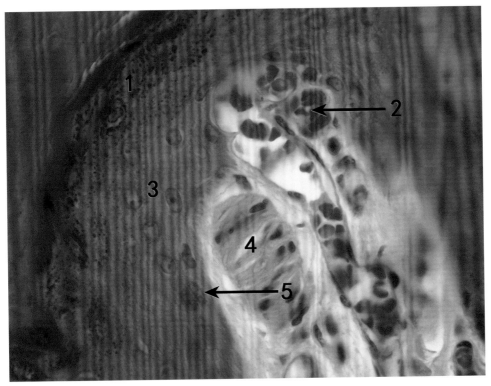

1. 颗粒层(stratum granulosum) 2. 毛细血管(capillary) 3. 棘层(stratum spinosum)

4. 触觉小体(tactile corpuscle) 5. 基底层(stratum basale)

图 11-3 触觉小体：人指皮(HE 染色，×100)

Pic. 11-3 Tactile corpuscle：Human finger skin. HE staining ×100

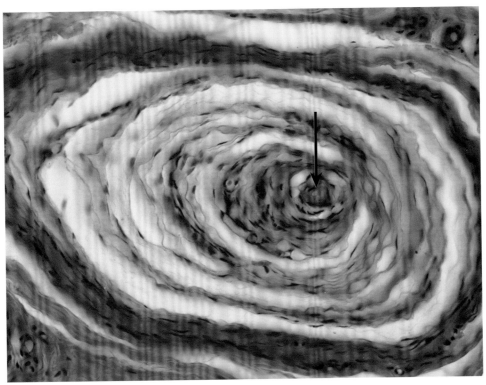

箭头示圆柱体。The arrow shows cylinder.

图 11-4 环层小体：人指皮(HE 染色，×100)

Pic. 11-4 Lamellar corpuscle：Human finger skin. HE staining ×100

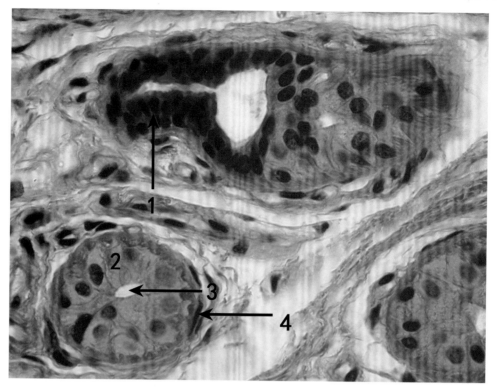

1.汗腺导管(duct of sweat gland) 2.汗腺分泌部(secretory portion of sweat gland)
3.腺腔(glandular lumen) 4.肌上皮细胞(myoepithelial cell)
图 11 - 5　汗腺:人指皮(HE 染色,×100)
Pic. 11 - 5　Sweat gland:Human finger skin. HE staining ×100

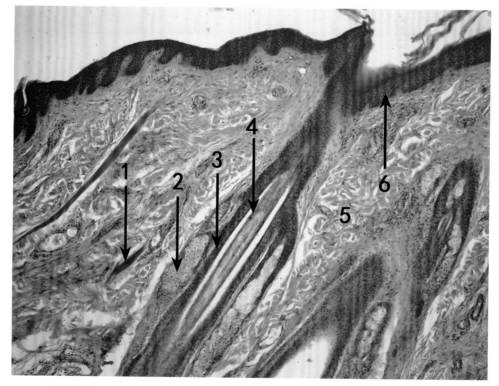

1.立毛肌(arrector pilli muscle) 2.皮脂腺(sebaceous gland) 3.毛囊(hair follicle)
4.毛根(hair root) 5.真皮(dermis) 6.表皮(epithelium)
图 11 - 6　头皮:人(HE 染色,×10)
Pic. 11 - 6　Scalp:Human. HE staining ×10

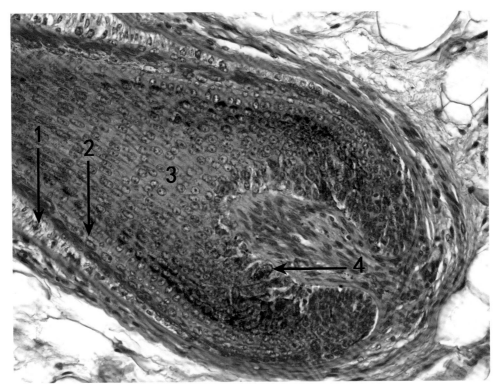

1.外根鞘(external root sheath) 2.内根鞘(internal root sheath) 3.毛根(hair root) 4.毛母质细胞(hair matrix cell)

图 11 - 7 毛球:人头皮(HE 染色,×100)

Pic. 11 - 7 Hair bulb:Human scalp. HE staining ×100

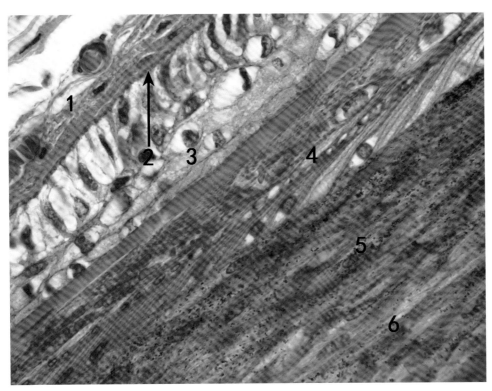

1.结缔组织鞘(connective tissue root sheath) 2.玻璃膜(glassy membrane) 3.外根鞘(external root sheath)

4.内根鞘(internal root sheath) 5.毛皮质(hair cortex) 6.毛髓质(hair medulla)

图 11 - 8 毛根纵断:人头皮(HE 染色,×100)

Pic. 11 - 8 Longitudinal section of hair root:Human scalp. HE staining ×100

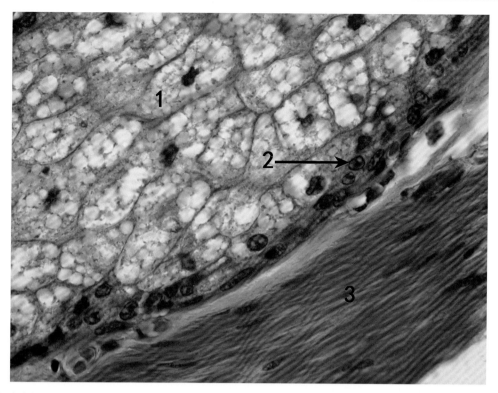

1. 皮脂腺成熟腺细胞（mature glandular cell of sebaceous gland） 2. 皮脂腺基细胞（basal cell of sebaceous gland）

3. 立毛肌（arrector pilli muscle）

图 11 - 9　皮脂腺和立毛肌：人头皮（HE 染色，×100）

Pic. 11 - 9　Sebaceous gland and arrector pili muscle：Human scalp. HE staining　×100

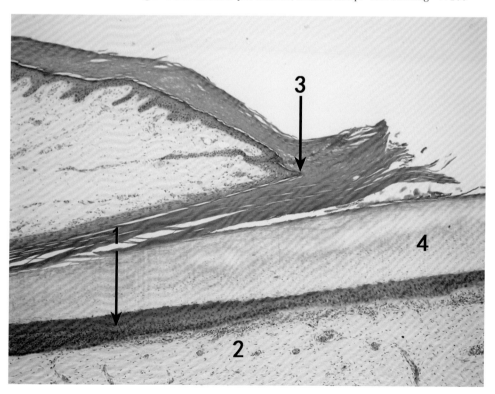

1. 甲床复层扁平上皮（stratified squamous epithelium of nail bed） 2. 甲床结缔组织（connective tissue of nail bed）

3. 甲襞（nail fold） 4. 甲体（nail body）

图 11 - 10　指甲：人（HE 染色，×100）

Pic. 11 - 10　Nail：Human. HE staining　×100

第十二章 消化管

实验基本要求:

1. 了解舌乳头、味蕾和牙的结构和功能。

2. 熟悉消化管壁的一般结构和功能。

3. 熟悉大肠和阑尾的结构特点和功能。

4. 掌握食管的组织结构特点。

5. 掌握胃底腺及其细胞组成类型、LM 和 EM 结构及功能。贲门腺和幽门腺的结构特点。

6. 掌握小肠黏膜及其上皮细胞的类型、LM 和 EM 结构及功能。小肠绒毛、小肠腺的形态结构。淋巴组织的分布及功能。

7. 光镜下能熟练识别消化管及其各段。

8. 相关超微结构和功能可通过课堂讨论等完成。

Chapter 12　Digestive tract

 Basic requirements for the experiment

1. Know the structures and functions of lingual papilla, taste bud and tooth.

2. Familiar with the general structures of the digestive tract wall.

3. Familiar with the structures and functions of large intestine and appendix.

4. Master the structural features of the esophagus.

5. Master the LM and EM structures and functions of gastric gland and the gland composition cells. The structural features of cardiac and pyloric gland.

6. Master the LM and EM structures and functions of intestinal mucosa and its composition epithelial cell. The morphology and structures of the villus and the intestinal gland. The distributions and functions of lymphoid tissue.

7. Identify different segments of digestive tract under LM.

8. The corresponding EM structures and functions will be discussed in lab.

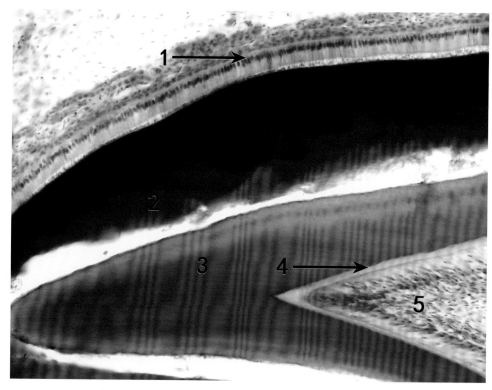

1.成釉质细胞(ameloblast) 2.牙釉质(enamel) 3.牙本质(dentin)
4.成牙本质细胞(odontoblast) 5.牙髓(dental pulp)
图 12 - 1 牙冠：人。磨片(HE 染色,×20)
Pic.12 - 1 Dental crown：Human. Ground section,HE staining ×20

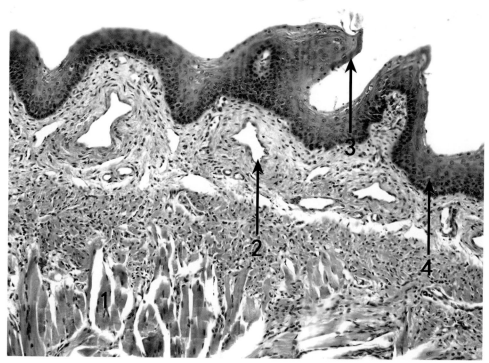

1.舌骨骼肌(skeletal muscle of tongue) 2.固有层血管(small blood vessel in lamina propria)
3.丝状乳头(filiform papilla) 4.黏膜上皮(mucosal epithelium)
图 12 - 2 舌：猫(HE 染色,×20)
Pic.12 - 2 Tongue：Cat. HE staining ×20

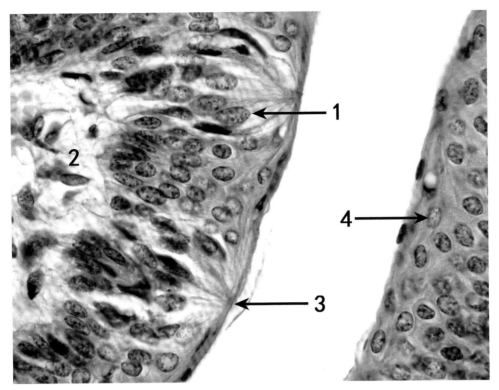

1.味细胞(taste cell)　2.固有层(lamina propria)　3.味孔(gustatory pore)

4.舌黏膜上皮(mucosal epithelium of tongue)

图 12-3　味蕾:猫(HE 染色,×100)

Pic. 12-3　Taste bud:Cat. HE staining　×100

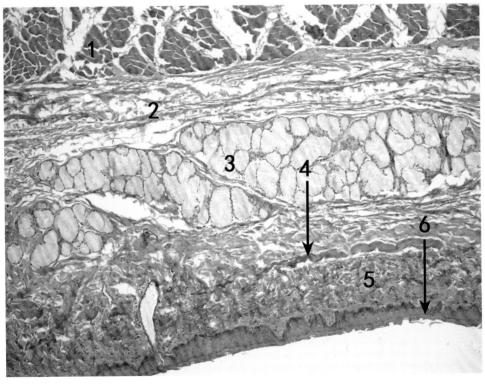

1.肌层(muscularis)　2.黏膜下层(submucosa)　3.黏膜下层内的混合腺体(mixed glands in submucosa)

4.黏膜肌层(muscularis mucosa)　5.固有层(lamina propria)　6.复层扁平上皮(stratified squamous epithelium)

图 12-4　食管:人(HE 染色,×10)

Pic. 12-4　Esophagus:Human. HE staining　×10

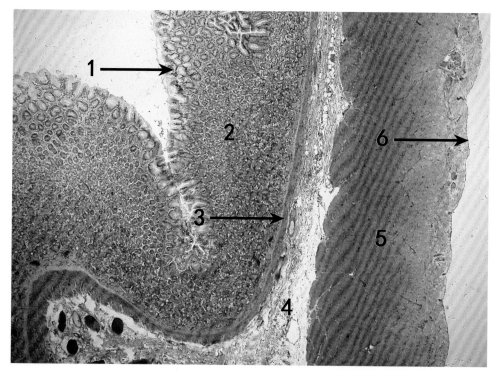

1. 黏膜上皮(mucosal epithelium) 2. 固有层(lamina propria) 3. 黏膜肌层(muscularis mucosa)

4. 黏膜下层(submucosa) 5. 肌层(muscularis) 6. 浆膜(serosa)

图 12-5 胃底:猫(HE 染色,×4)

Pic. 12-5 Fundus of stomach:Cat. HE staining ×4

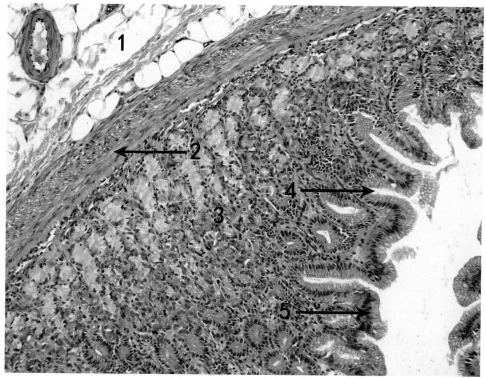

1. 黏膜下层(submucosa) 2. 黏膜肌层(muscularis mucosa) 3. 胃底腺(fundic glands)

4. 胃小凹(gastric pit) 5. 黏膜上皮(mucosal epithelium)

图 12-6 胃底黏膜:猫(HE 染色,×20)

Pic. 12-6 Fundic mucosa:Cat. HE staining ×20

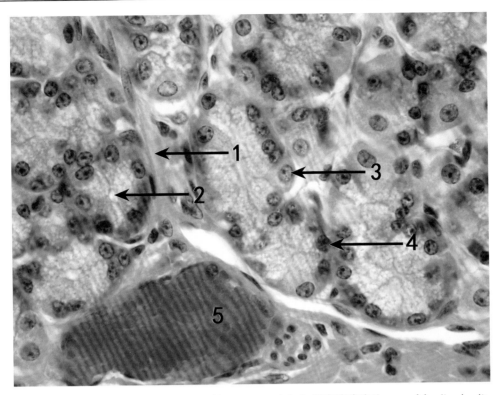

1.固有层结缔组织（connective tissue of lamina propria）　2.胃底腺腺腔（lumen of fundic gland）

3.壁细胞（parietal cell）　4.主细胞（chief cell）　5.小血管（small blood vessel）

图 12-7　胃底腺：猫（HE 染色，×100）

Pic. 12-7　Fundic gland：Cat. HE staining　×100

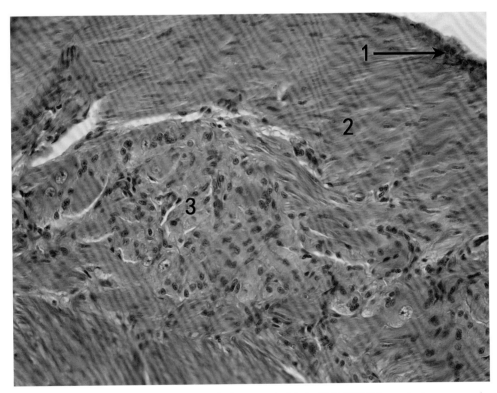

1.浆膜（serosa）　2.肌层平滑肌（smooth muscle in muscularis）　3.肌间神经丛（myenteric nervous plexus）

图 12-8　肌间神经丛：猫胃底（HE 染色，×40）

Pic. 12-8　Myenteric nerve plexus：Cat fundus. HE staining　×40

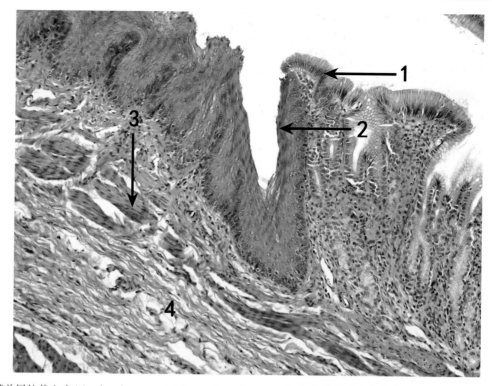

1.胃黏膜单层柱状上皮（simple columnar epithelium of gastric mucosa）2.食管黏膜未角化复层扁平上皮（nonkeratinized stratified squamous epithelium of esophageal mucosa）3.黏膜肌层（muscularis mucosa）4.黏膜下层（submucosa）

图 12 - 9　胃贲门：猫（HE 染色，×20）

Pic. 12 - 9　Cardia of stomach：Cat. HE staining　×20

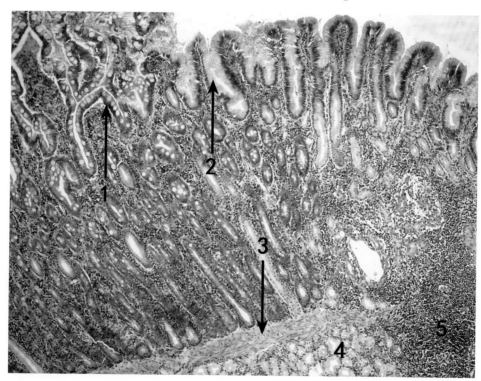

1.十二指肠黏膜单层柱状上皮（simple columnar epithelium of duodenal mucosa）2.胃黏膜单层柱状上皮（simple columnar epithelium of gastric mucosa）3.黏膜肌层（muscularis mucosa）4.十二指肠腺（duodenal glands）5.淋巴组织（lymphoid tissue）

图 12 - 10　胃幽门：猫（HE 染色，×20）

Pic. 12 - 10　Pylorus of stomach：Cat. HE staining　×20

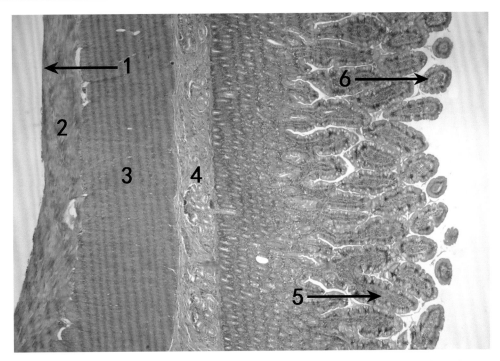

1. 浆膜（serosa）　2. 肌层的外纵肌（external longitudinal muscle of muscularis）　3. 肌层的内环层肌（internal circular muscle of muscularis）　4. 十二指肠腺（duodenal glands）　5. 绒毛纵断面（longitudinal section of a villus）　6. 绒毛横断面（cross section of a villus）

图 12 - 11　十二指肠：猫（HE 染色，×4）

Pic. 12 - 11　Duodenum：Cat. HE staining　×4

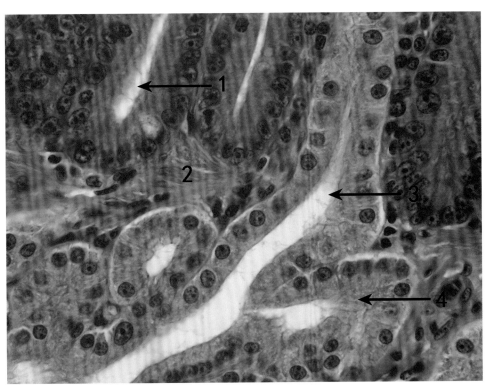

1. 小肠腺（small intestinal gland）　2. 黏膜肌层（muscularis mucosa）　3. 十二指肠腺导管（duct of duodenal gland）

4. 十二指肠腺分泌部（secretory portion of duodenal gland）

图 12 - 12　十二指肠腺：猫（HE 染色，×100）

Pic. 12 - 12　Duodenal gland：Cat. HE staining　×100

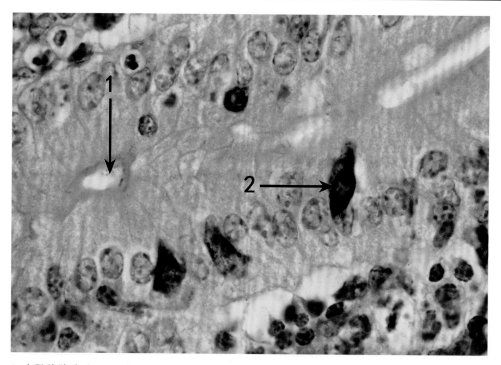

1. 小肠腺腺腔（lumen of small intestinal gland） 2. 小肠腺上皮内的内分泌细胞（endocrine cell in epithelium of small intestinal gland）

图 12 - 13　内分泌细胞：猫十二指肠（银染，×100）

Pic. 12 - 13　Endocrine cells：Cat duodenum. Silver staining　×100

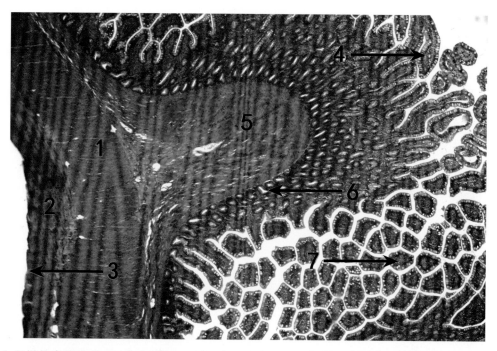

1. 肌层的内环肌（internal circular muscle of muscularis） 2. 肌层的外纵肌（external longitudinal muscle of muscularis） 3. 浆膜（serosa） 4. 绒毛纵断面（longitudinal section of a villus） 5. 黏膜下层（submucosa） 6. 小肠腺（small intestinal gland） 7. 绒毛横断面（cross section of a villus）

图 12 - 14　空肠：猫（HE 染色，×4）

Pic. 12 - 14　Jejunum：Cat. HE staining　×4

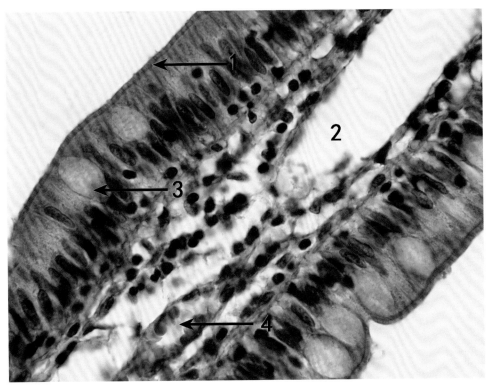

1.纹状缘(striated border)　2.中央乳糜管(central lacteal)　3.杯状细胞(goblet cell)

4.固有层内的毛细血管(capillary in lamina propria)

图 12－15　肠绒毛：猫空肠(HE 染色,×100)

Pic.12－15　Intestinal villus：Cat jejunum. HE staining　×100

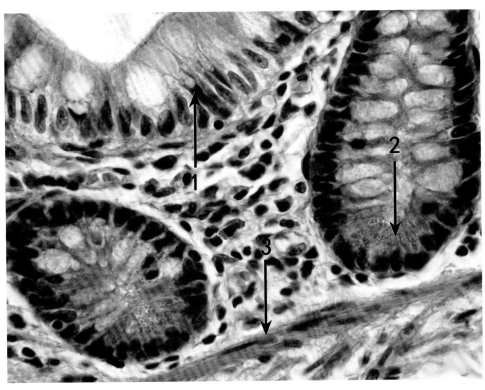

1.肠黏膜上皮(mucosal epithelium of intestine)　2.小肠腺底部的帕内特细胞(Paneth cells in basal portion of small intestinal gland)　3.黏膜肌层(muscularis mucosa)

图 12－16　帕内特细胞：猫空肠(HE 染色,×100)

Pic.12－16　Paneth cell：Cat jejunum. HE staining　×100

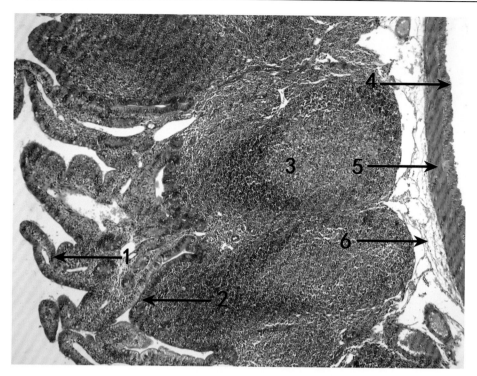

1.绒毛(villus) 2.覆盖在固有层内淋巴小结表面的黏膜上皮(mucosal epithelium covering lymphoid nodule in lamina propria) 3.集合淋巴小结(aggregated lymphoid nodules) 4.浆膜(serosa) 5.肌层(muscularis) 6.黏膜下层(submucosa)

图 12 - 17 回肠:猫(HE 染色,×10)

Pic. 12 - 17 Ileum:Cat. HE staining ×10

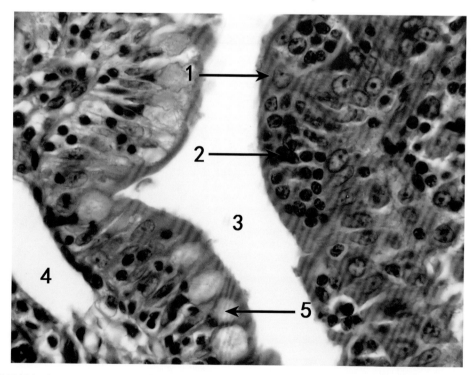

1.微皱褶细胞(microfold cell) 2.微皱褶细胞底部内包含的多个淋巴细胞和巨噬细胞等(lymphocytes, macrophages and other cells enveloped by basal pit of microfold cell) 3.回肠肠腔(ileal lumen) 4.中央乳糜管(central lacteal) 5.杯状细胞(goblet cell)

图 12 - 18 微皱褶细胞:猫回肠(HE 染色,×100)

Pic. 12 - 18 Microfold cell:Cat ileum. HE staining ×100

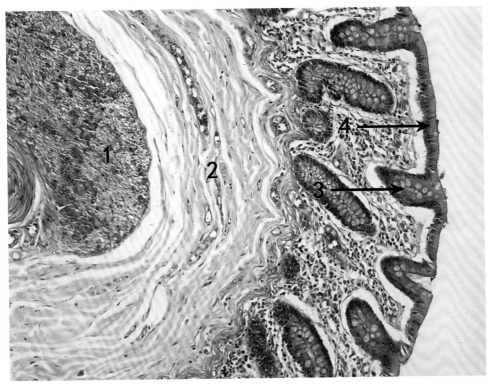

1.肌层(muscularis)　2.黏膜下层(submucosa)　3.大肠腺(large intestinal gland)

4.黏膜上皮(mucosal epithelium)

图 12-19　结肠:猫(HE 染色,×10)

Pic. 12-19　Colon:Cat. HE staining　×10

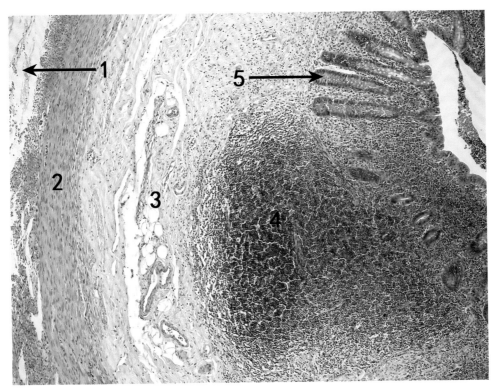

1.外膜(adventitia)　2.肌层(muscularis)　3.黏膜下层(submucosa)　4.固有层和黏膜下层内的淋巴组织

(lymphatic tissue in lamina propria and submucosa)　5.大肠腺(large intestinal gland)

图 12-20　阑尾:人(HE 染色,×10)

Pic. 12-20　Appendix:Human. HE staining　×10

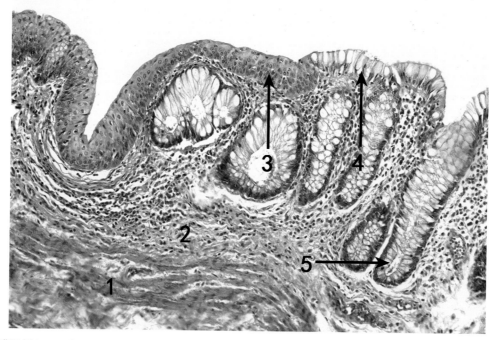

1. 黏膜肌层（muscularis mucosa） 2. 固有层（lamina propria） 3. 复层扁平上皮（stratified squamous epithelium）
4. 单层柱状上皮（simple columnar epithelium） 5. 大肠腺（large intestinal gland）

图 12 - 21　直肠-肛管交界处：人（HE 染色，×20）

Pic. 12 - 21　Recto-anal junction：Human. HE staining　×20

第十三章　消化腺

实验基本要求：

1. 了解大唾液腺的一般结构。熟悉浆液性、黏液性和混合性腺泡的结构特点。

2. 熟悉胆囊的结构特点。

3. 掌握胰腺的一般结构。外分泌部的 LM 和 EM 结构和功能，内分泌部胰岛的结构特点以及各类胰岛细胞的分类和功能。

4. 掌握肝的一般结构。肝小叶、肝细胞、肝血窦、窦周隙、胆小管的 LM 和 EM 结构及功能。肝门管区的结构。

5. 光镜下识别肝、胰腺和胆囊。

6. 相关超微结构和功能可通过课堂讨论等完成。

Chapter 13　Digestive gland

 Basic requirements for the experiment

1. Know the general structures of large salivary gland. Familiar with the structural features of serous acini, mucous acini and mixed acini.

2. Familiar with the general structures of gallbladder.

3. Master the general structures of pancreas. The LM and EM structures and functions of exocrine part, structural features of endocrine part, the pancreas islet, and classifications and functions of endocrine cell.

4. Master the general structures of liver. The LM and EM structures and functions of hepatic lobule, hepatocyte, sinusoid, perisinusoidal space and bile canaliculus. The structures of portal area.

5. Identify pancreas, liver and gallbladder under LM.

6. The corresponding EM structures and functions will be discussed in lab.

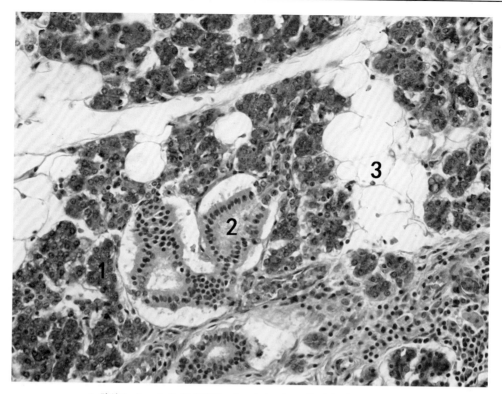

1.腺泡(acinus) 2.纹状管(striated duct) 3.脂肪细胞(adipocyte)

图 13-1 腮腺：人(HE 染色，×40)

Pic.13-1 Parotid gland：Human. HE staining ×40

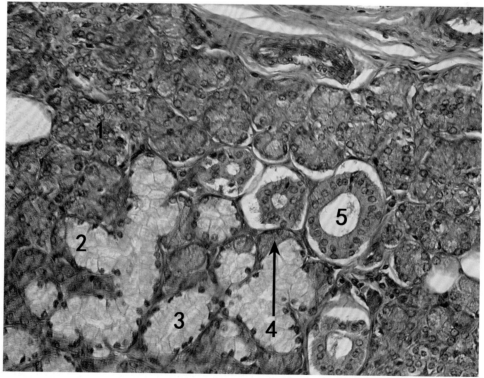

1.浆液性腺泡(serous acinus) 2.混合性腺泡(mixed acinus) 3.黏液性腺泡(mucous acinus)

4.浆半月(serous demilune) 5.纹状管(striated duct)

图 13-2 下颌下腺：人(HE 染色，×40)

Pic.13-2 Submandibular gland：Human. HE staining ×40

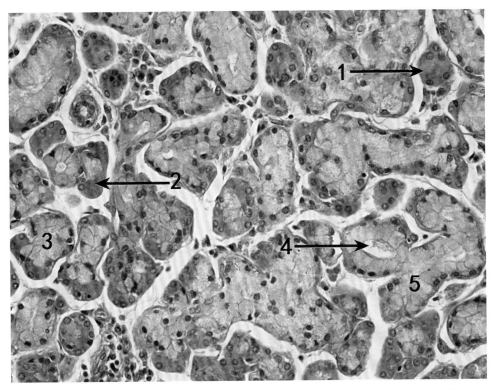

1. 浆液性腺泡（serous acinus）　2. 浆半月（serous demilune）　3. 混合性腺泡（mixed acinus）　4. 腺泡腔（acinar lumen）

5. 黏液性腺泡（mucous acinus）

图 13 - 3　舌下腺：人（HE 染色，×40）

Pic. 13 - 3　Sublingual gland：Human. HE staining　×40

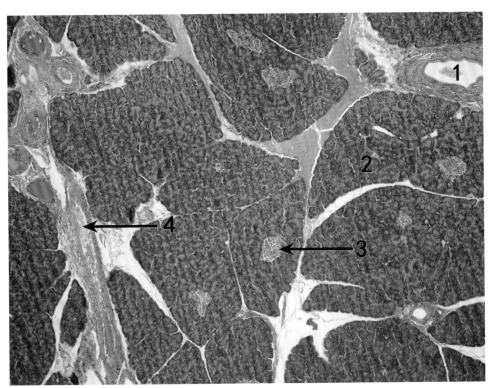

1. 小叶间导管（interlobular duct）　2. 外分泌部（exocrine portion）　3. 胰岛（pancreas islet）

4. 小叶间结缔组织中的小血管（small blood vessel in interlobular connective tissue）

图 13 - 4　胰腺：人（HE 染色，×10）

Pic. 13 - 4　Pancreas：Human. HE staining　×10

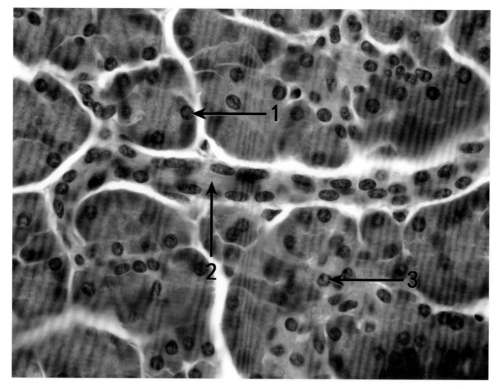

1.腺泡细胞(acinar cell) 2.闰管(intercalated duct) 3.泡心细胞(centroacinar cell)

图 13－5　胰腺腺泡:人(HE 染色,×100)

Pic. 13－5　Pancreatic acinus:Human. HE staining　×100

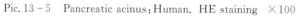

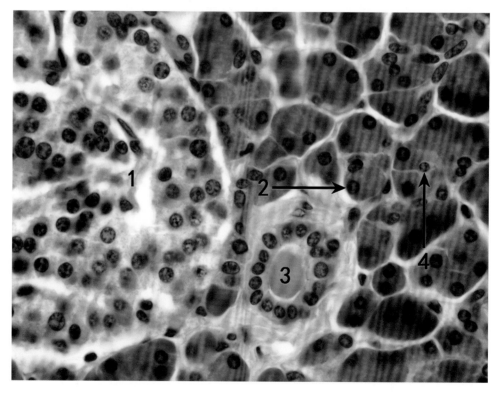

1.胰岛(pancreas islet) 2.腺泡细胞(acinar cell) 3.小叶内导管(intralobular duct) 4.泡心细胞(centroacinar cell)

图 13－6　胰岛:人(HE 染色,×100)

Pic. 13－6　Pancreas islet:Human. HE staining　×100

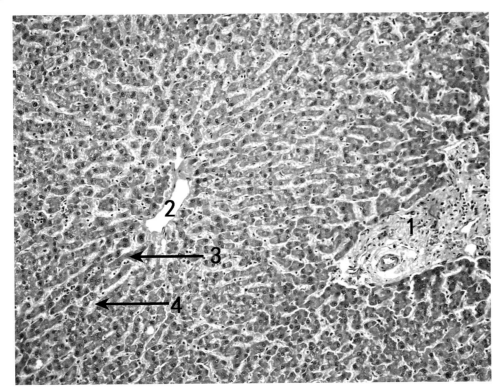

1.门管区(portal area) 2.中央静脉(central vein) 3.肝板(hepatic plate) 4.肝血窦(hepatic sinusoid)

图 13-7 肝小叶:人(HE 染色,×20)

Pic. 13-7 Hepatic lobule:Human. HE staining ×20

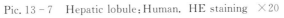

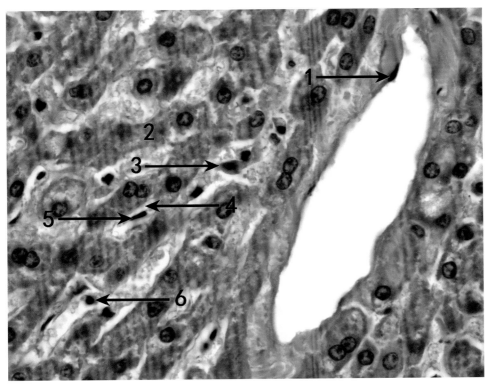

1.中央静脉内皮(endothelium of central vein) 2.肝板(hepatic plate) 3.肝血窦内的肝巨噬细胞(hepatic macrophage in hepatic sinusoid) 4.肝窦周隙(perisinusoidal space) 5.血窦内皮(endothelium of sinusoid) 6.肝血窦内的淋巴细胞(lymphocyte in hepatic sinusoid)

图 13-8 肝小叶:人(HE 染色,×100)

Pic. 13-8 Hepatic lobule:Human. HE staining ×100

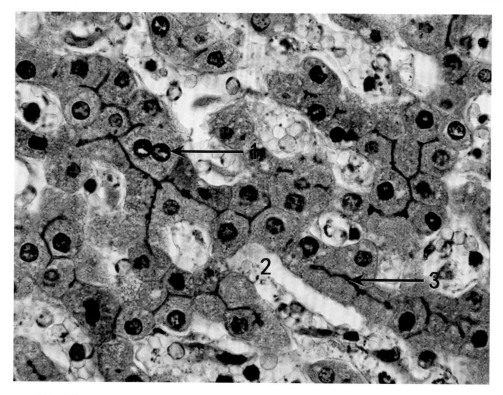

1. 肝细胞核(nuclei of a hepatocyte) 2. 肝血窦(hepatic sinusoid) 3. 胆小管(bile canaliculus)

图 13 - 9   胆小管：人(铁苏木素染色，×100)

Pic. 13 - 9   Bile canaliculus：Human. Iron-hematoxylin staining   ×100

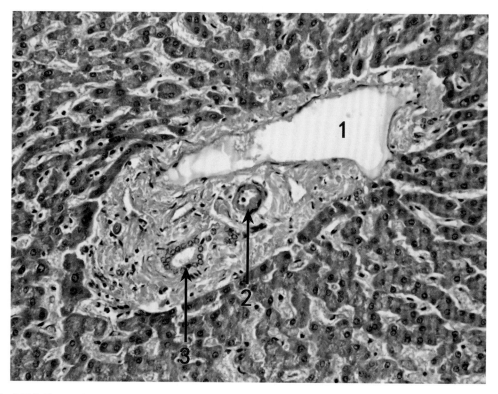

1. 小叶间静脉(interlobular vein) 2. 小叶间动脉(interlobular artery) 3. 小叶间胆管(interlobular bile duct)

图 13 - 10   门管区：人(HE 染色，×40)

Pic. 13 - 10   Portal area：Human. HE staining   ×40

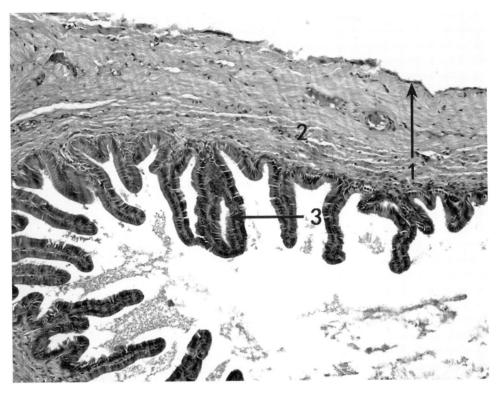

1.外膜(serosa) 2.肌层(muscularis) 3.黏膜隆起(mucosal fold)

图 13 - 11 胆囊：人(HE 染色,×20)

Pic. 13 - 11 Gall bladder：Human. HE staining ×20

第十四章 呼吸系统

实验基本要求：

1. 熟悉呼吸系统的组成和功能。

2. 掌握肺的一般结构。肺导气部各段、呼吸部各段的结构特点和变化规律；两种肺泡细胞的微细结构；肺泡隔、肺巨噬细胞和肺泡孔的结构和功能。

3. 掌握气管和支气管的组织结构与功能。

4. 光镜下识别气管、支气管、小支气管、终末细支气管、呼吸性细支气管、肺泡管和肺泡。

5. 相关超微结构和功能可通过课堂讨论等完成。

Chapter 14　Respiratory System

 Basic requirements for the experiment

1. Familiar with the compositions and functions of the respiratory system.

2. Master the general structures of lung. The structural features and changing pattern of different segments of conducting and respiratory portions. The structure and functions of type Ⅰ and Ⅱ alveolar cell. The structures and functions of interalveolar septum, alveolar macrophage and alveolar pore.

3. Master the structures and functions of the trachea and bronchus.

4. Identify trachea, bronchus, bronchiole, terminal bronchiole, respiratory bronchiole, alveolar duct and alveolus under LM.

5. The corresponding EM structures and functions will be discussed in lab.

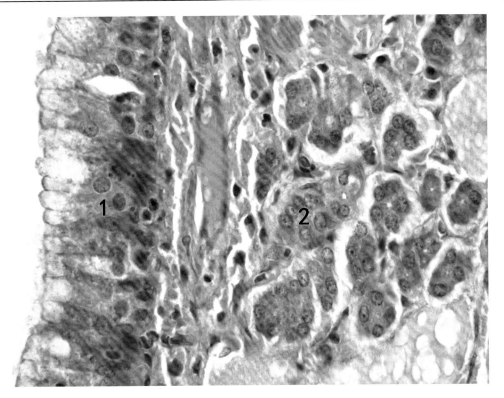

1. 嗅上皮（olfactory epithelium）　2. 固有层中的浆液性嗅腺（serous olfactory glands in lamina propria）

图 14 – 1　嗅上皮：兔（HE 染色，×100）

Pic. 14 – 1　Olfactory epithelium：Rabbit. HE staining　×100

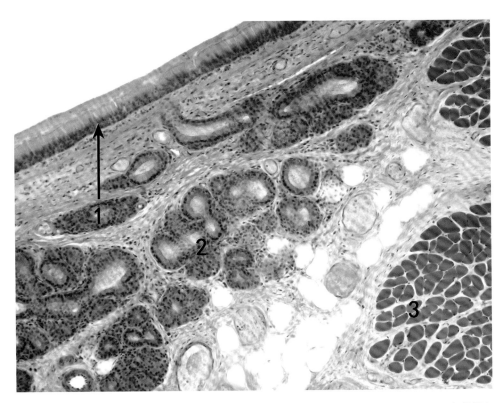

1. 黏膜上皮（mucosal epithelium）　2. 固有层中的混合腺体（mixed glands in lamina propria）　3. 声带肌（vocalis）

图 14 – 2　喉室壁：猫（HE 染色，×20）

Pic. 14 – 2　Ventricular fold of larynx：Cat. HE staining　×20

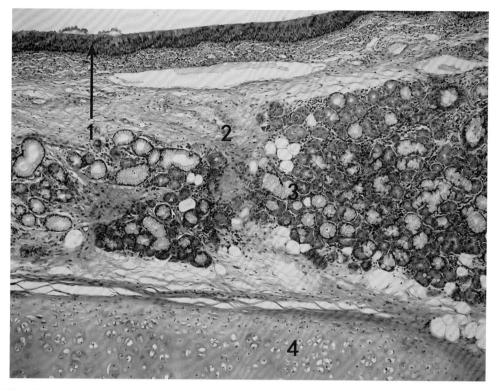

1. 黏膜上皮(mucosal epithelium) 2. 固有层(lamina propria) 3. 黏膜下层的混合性气管腺(mixed tracheal glands in submucosa) 4. 外膜中的透明软骨(hyaline cartilage in adventitia)

图 14 - 3　气管：人(HE 染色，×10)

Pic. 14 - 3　Trachea：Human. HE staining　×10

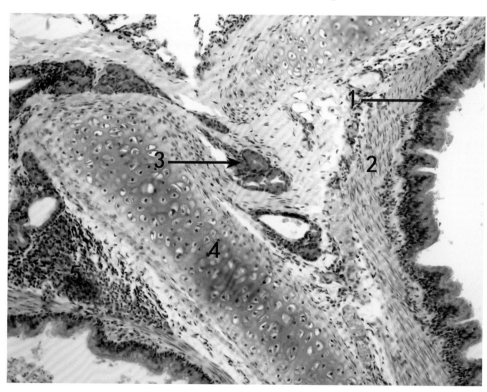

1. 黏膜上皮(mucosal epithelium) 2. 固有层中的平滑肌(smooth muscle in lamina propria) 3. 黏膜下层的腺体(glands in submucosa) 4. 外膜中的透明软骨片(hyaline cartilage plate in adventitia) 5. 淋巴组织(lymphoid tissue)

图14-4　小支气管：人(HE 染色，×20)

Pic. 14 - 4　Small bronchus：Human. HE staining　×20

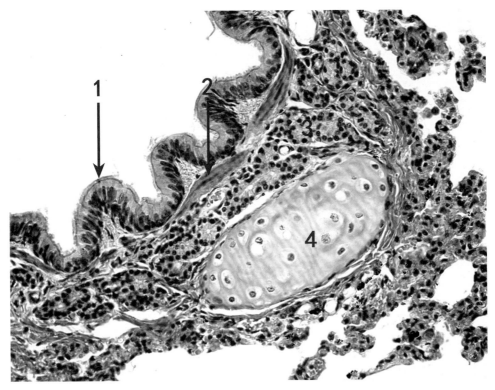

1.黏膜上皮(mucosal epithelium) 2.固有层的平滑肌(smooth muscle in lamina propria)

3.黏膜下层的腺体(glands in submucosa) 4.外膜中的软骨片(hyaline cartilage plate in adventitia)

图 14 - 5 细支气管：人(HE 染色，×100)

Pic. 14 - 5 Bronchiole：Human. HE staining ×100

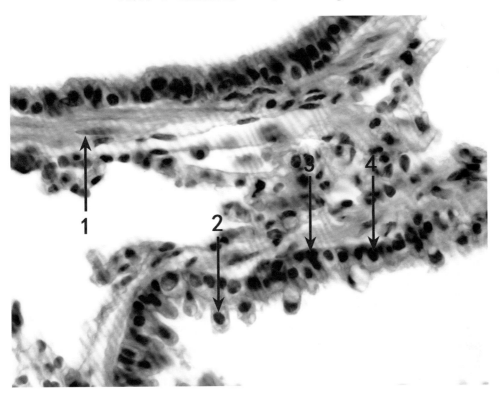

1.平滑肌(smooth muscle) 2.克拉拉细胞(Clara cell) 3.单层柱状细胞(simple columnar epithelium)

4.纤毛细胞(ciliated cell)

图 14-6 终末细支气管：人(HE 染色，×100)

Pic. 14-6 Terminal bronchiole：Human. HE staining ×100

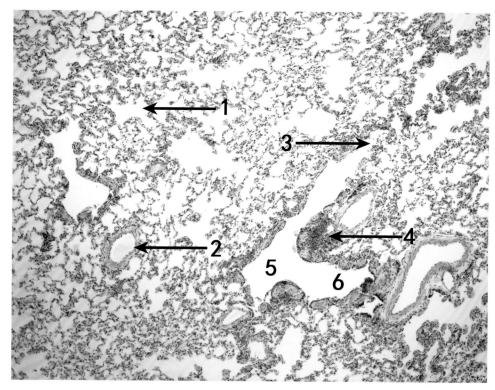

1.肺泡囊（alveolar sac） 2.肺动脉分支（branch of pulmonary artery） 3.肺泡管（alveolar duct） 4.肺黏膜相关淋巴组织（mucosa-associated lymphoid tissue in lung） 5.呼吸性细支气管（respiratory bronchiole） 6.终末细支气管（terminal bronchiole）

图 14－7　肺呼吸部：人（HE 染色，×10）

Pic. 14－7　Respiratory portion of lung：Human. HE staining　×10

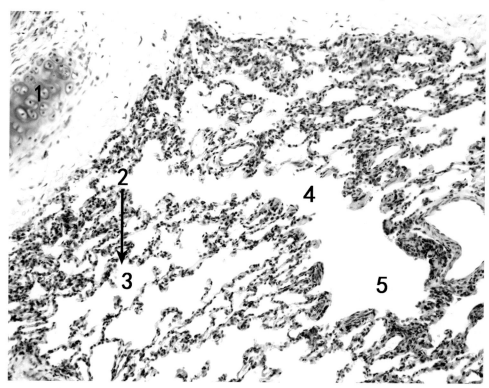

1.透明软骨片（hyaline cartilage plate） 2.肺泡（alveolus） 3.肺泡囊（alveolar sac）

4.肺泡管（alveolar duct） 5.呼吸性细支气管（respiratory bronchiole）

图 14－8　肺呼吸部：人（HE 染色，×20）

Pic. 14－8　Respiratory portion of lung：Human. HE staining　×20

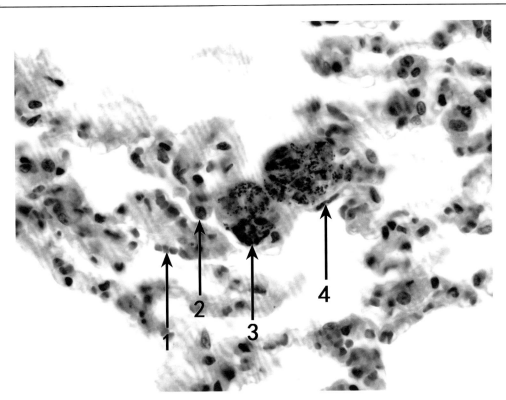

1.肺泡隔内的毛细血管（capillary in alveolar septum）　2.Ⅱ型肺泡细胞（type Ⅱ alveolar cell）

3.尘细胞（dust cells）　4.Ⅰ型肺泡细胞（type Ⅰ alveolar cell）

图 14 - 9　肺泡：人（HE 染色，×100）

Pic. 14 - 9　Pulmonary alveolus：Human. HE staining　×100

第十五章　泌尿系统

实验基本要求：

1.了解泌尿系统的组成和功能。

2.熟悉肾的一般结构。掌握肾小体、肾小管各段的 LM 和 EM 结构与功能。集合管的结构特点和功能；球旁复合体的组成、结构和功能。

3.熟悉输尿管、膀胱和尿道的结构。

4.光镜下识别肾和膀胱。

5.相关超微结构和功能可通过课堂讨论等完成。

Chapter 15　Urinary system

 Basic requirements for the experiment

1. Know the compositions and functions of urinary system.

2. Familiar with the general structures of kidney. Master the LM and EM structures and functions of nephron, renal corpuscle, uriniferous tubule and collecting duct. The compositions, structures and functions of juxtaglomerular apparatus.

3. Familiar with the structures of ureter, urinary bladder and urethra.

4. Identify kidney and urinary bladder under LM.

5. The corresponding EM structures and functions will be discussed in lab.

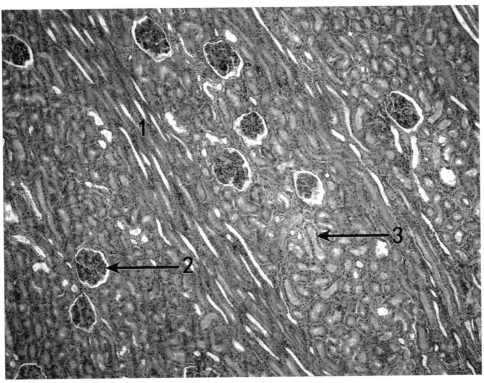

1.髓放线（medullary ray） 2.肾小体（renal corpuscle） 3.皮质迷路内的肾小管（renal tubule in cortical labyrinth）

图 15 - 1　肾皮质：人（HE 染色，×10）

Pic. 15 - 1　Renal cortex：Human. HE staining　×10

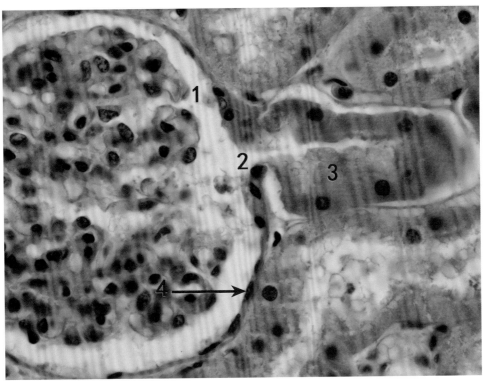

1.肾小囊腔（capsular space） 2.尿极（urinary pole）.3 近曲小管（proximal convoluted tubule）

4.肾小囊壁层（parietal layer of renal capsule）

图 15 - 2　肾小体尿极：人（HE 染色，×100）

Pic. 15 - 2　Urinary pole of renal corpuscle：Human. HE staining　×100

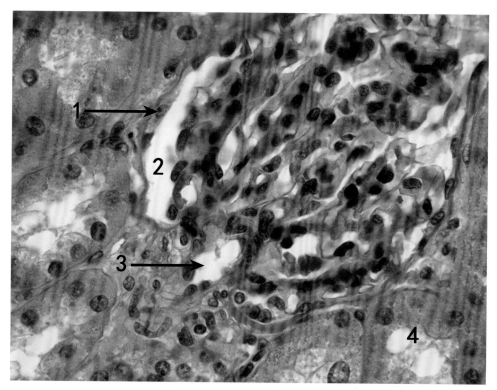

1. 肾小囊壁层(parietal layer of renal capsule) 2. 肾小囊腔(capsular space) 3. 血管极(vascular pole)

4. 近曲小管(proximal convoluted tubule)

图 15-3　肾小体血管极：人（HE 染色，×100）

Pic. 15-3　Vascular pole of renal corpuscle：Human. HE staining　×100

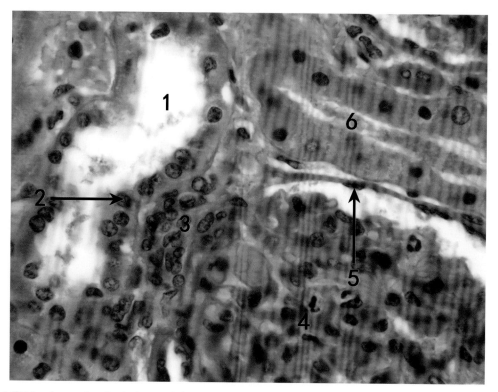

1. 远曲小管(distal convoluted tubule) 2. 致密斑(macula densa) 3. 球外系膜细胞(extraglomerular mesangial cells)

4. 肾小体(renal corpuscle) 5. 肾小囊壁层(parietal layer of renal capsule) 6. 近曲小管(proximal convoluted tubule)

图 15-4　致密斑：人（HE 染色，×100）

Pic. 15-4　Macula densa：Human. HE staining　×100

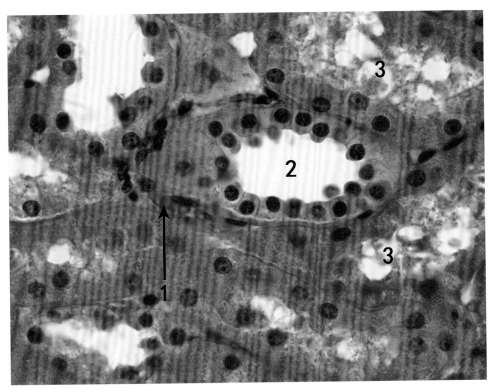

1. 毛细血管（capillary） 2. 远曲小管（distal convoluted tubule） 3. 近曲小管（proximal convoluted tubule）

图 15 - 5 近曲小管和远曲小管：人（HE 染色，×100）

Pic. 15 - 5 Proximal convoluted tubule and distal convoluted tubule：Human. HE staining ×100

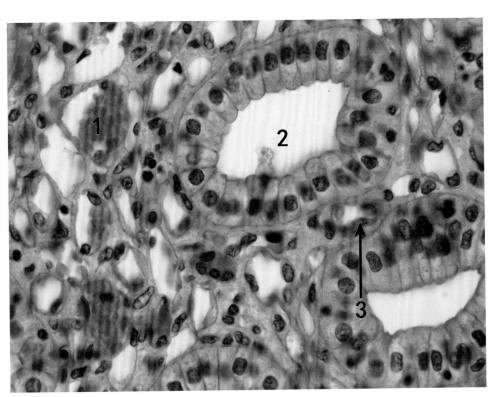

1. 小血管（small blood vessel） 2. 集合管（collecting duct） 3. 细段（thin segment）

图 15 - 6 肾髓质：人（HE 染色，×100）

Pic. 15 - 6 Renal medulla：Human. HE staining ×100

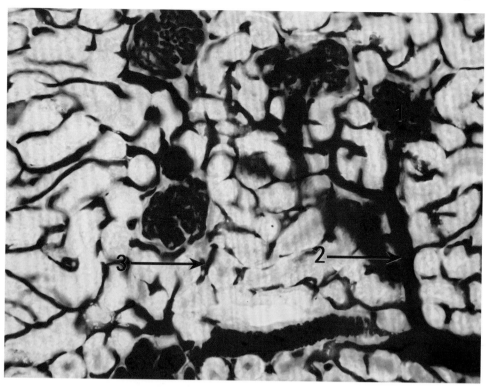

1. 血管球(glomerulus) 2. 小叶间动脉(interlobular artery) 3. 球后毛细血管网(postglomerular capillary)

图 15 - 7　肾血管:兔肾皮质(卡红明胶灌注,×40)

Pic. 15 - 7　Renal blood vessel:Rabbit renal cortex. Carmine red-gelatin perfusion　×40

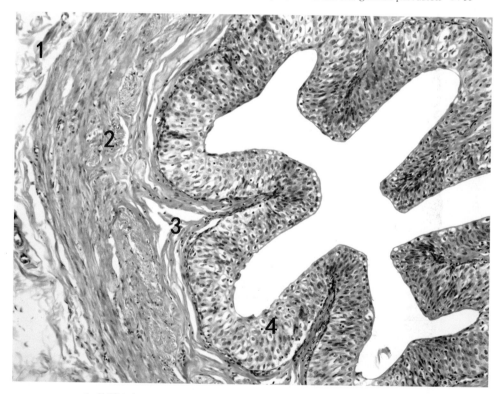

1. 外膜(adventitia) 2. 肌层(muscularis) 3. 固有层(lamina propria)

4. 黏膜上皮/变移上皮(mucosal epithelium/transitional epithelium)

图 15 - 8　输尿管:人(HE 染色,×20)

Pic. 15 - 8　Ureter:Human. HE staining　×20

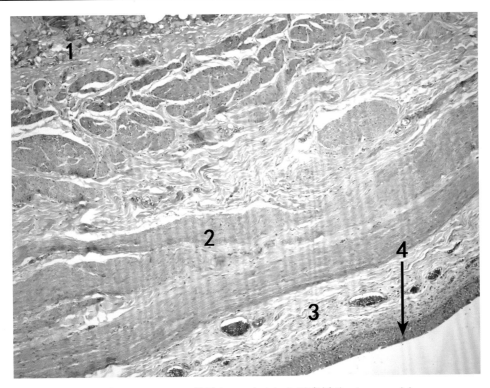

1. 外膜（adventitia）　2. 肌层（muscularis）　3. 固有层（lamina propria）

4. 黏膜上皮／变移上皮（mucosal epithelium/transitional epithelium）

图 15-9　膀胱：猫（HE 染色，×10）

Pic. 15-9　Urinary bladder：Cat. HE staining　×10

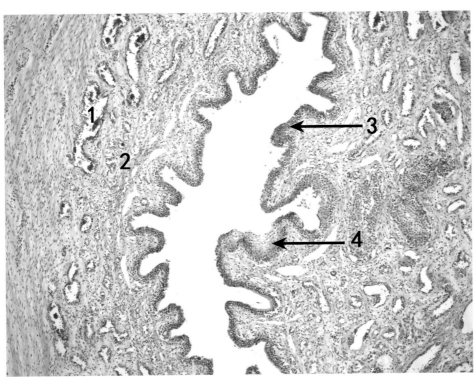

1. 尿道海绵体血窦（vascular space of corpus spongiosum）　2. 尿道黏膜固有层（lamina propria of urethral mucosa）　3. 尿道黏膜复层扁平上皮（stratified squamous epithelium of urethral mucosa）　4. 尿道黏膜假复层柱状上皮（pseudostratified columnar epithelium of urethral mucosa）

图 15-10　男性尿道海绵体部：人（HE 染色，×10）

Pic. 15-10　Cavernous part of male urethra：Human. HE staining　×10

第十六章 男性生殖系统

实验基本要求：

  1.了解男性生殖系统的组成和功能。

  2.了解前列腺和精囊的结构与功能。

  3.熟悉附睾和输精管的结构与功能。

  4.掌握睾丸和生精小管的结构特点。掌握各级生精细胞、支持细胞和间质细胞的形态、结构和功能。

  5.光镜下识别睾丸、精子、附睾、前列腺和精囊。

  6.相关超微结构和功能可通过课堂讨论等完成。

Chapter 16 Male reproductive system

 Basic requirements for the experiment

  1. Know the compositions and functions of male reproductive system.

  2. Know the structures and functions of prostate and seminal vesicle.

  3. Familiar with the structures and functions of epidydimis and ductus deferens.

  4. Master the structural features of testis and seminiferous tubule. Master the morphology, structures and functions of spermatogenic cell, sustentacular cell and interstitial cell.

  5. Identify testis, sperm, epidydimis, prostate and seminal vesicle under LM.

  6. The corresponding EM structures and functions will be discussed in lab.

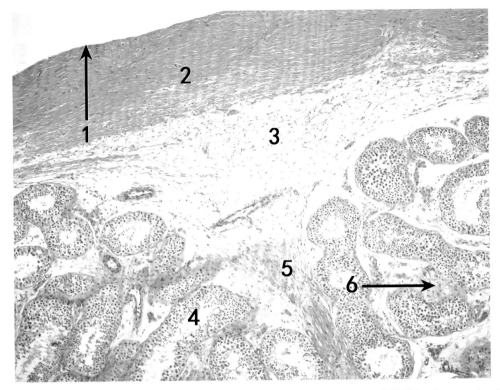

1.鞘膜脏层(visceral layer of tunica vaginalis) 2.白膜(tunica albuginea) 3.血管膜(tunica vasculosa)
4.生精小管(seminiferous tubule) 5.睾丸间隔(testis septum) 6.间质细胞(interstitial cell)

图 16-1 睾丸：人(HE 染色，×10)

Pic. 16-1 Testis：Human. HE staining ×10

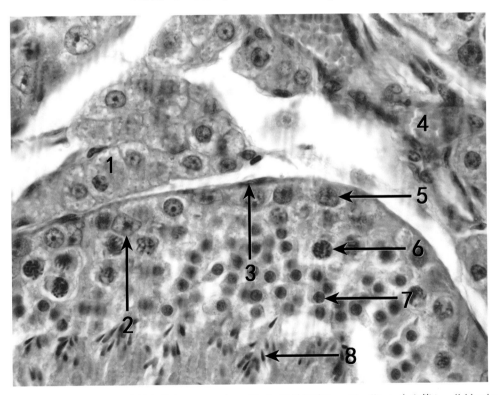

1.间质细胞(interstitial cell) 2.支持细胞(sustentacular cell) 3.肌样细胞(myoid cell) 4.小血管(small blood vessel)

5.精原细胞(spermatogonium) 6.初级精母细胞(primary spermatocyte) 7.精子细胞(spermatid) 8.精子(spermatozoon)

图 16-2 生精小管：人(HE 染色，×100)

Pic. 16-2 Seminiferous tubule：Human. HE staining ×100

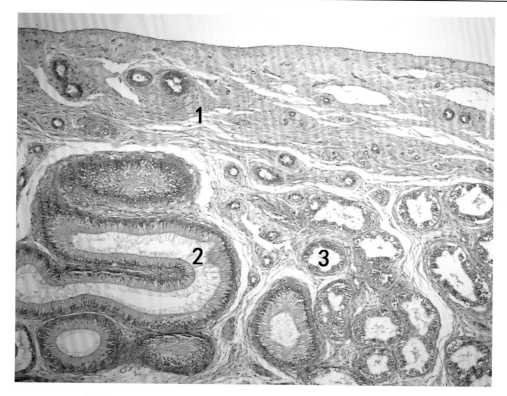

1. 被膜（capsule） 2. 附睾管（epididymal duct） 3. 输出小管（efferent duct）

图 16-3　输出小管和附睾管：人（HE 染色，×10）

Pic. 16-3　Efferent duct and epididymal duct：Human. HE staining　×10

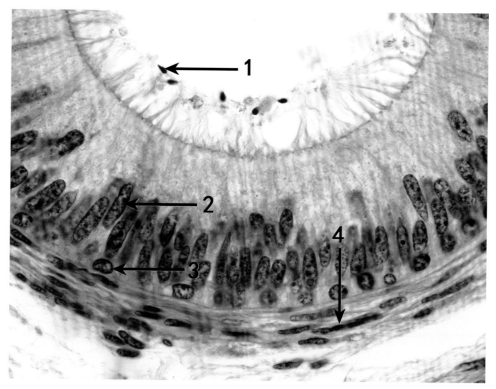

1. 精子（spermatozoon） 2. 主细胞（principal cell） 3. 基细胞（basal cell） 4. 平滑肌纤维（smooth muscle fiber）

图 16-4　附睾管：人（HE 染色，×100）

Pic. 16-4　Epididymal duct：Human. HE staining　×100

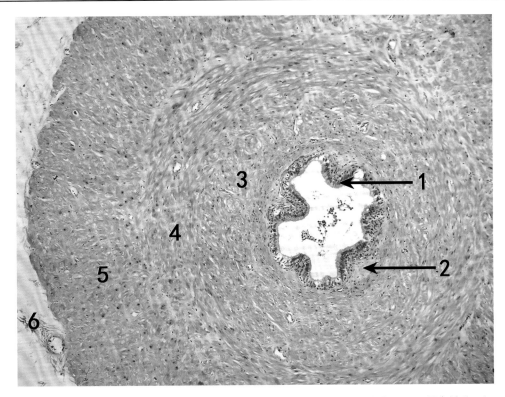

1. 黏膜上皮/假复层柱状上皮（mucosal epithelium/pseudostratified columnar epithelium）　2. 固有层（lamina propria）

3. 肌层的内纵肌（inner longitudinal muscle of muscularis）　4. 肌层的中环肌（middle circular muscle of muscularis）

5. 肌层的外纵肌（outer longitudinal muscle of muscularis）　6. 外膜（adventitia）

图 16－5　输精管：人（HE 染色，×10）

Pic. 16－5　Ductus deferens：Human. HE staining　×10

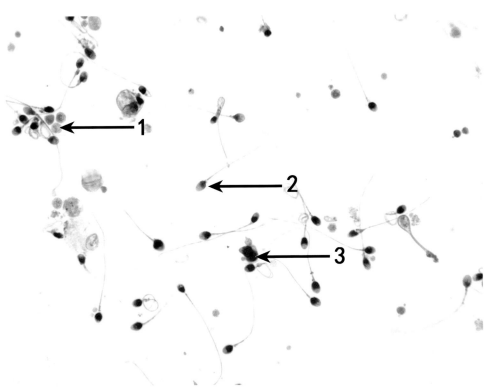

1. 脱落细胞（shed cell）　2. 正常精子（normal spermatozoon）　3. 异常精子（abnormal spermatozoon）

图 16－6　精子：人（精液涂片 HE 染色，×100）

Pic. 16－6　Spermatozoon：Human. Semen smear. HE staining　×100

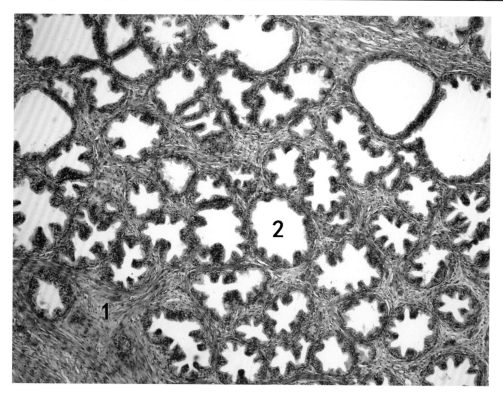

1. 被膜及其分支（capsule and its branches）　2. 腺腔（glandular lumen）

图 16 - 7　前列腺：人（HE 染色，×10）

Pic. 16 - 7　Prostate：Human. HE staining　×10

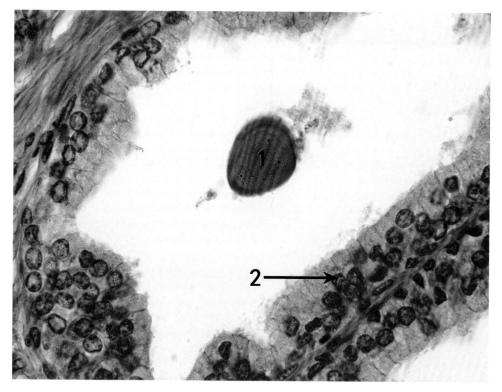

1. 前列腺凝固体（prostatic concretion）　2. 腺上皮（glandular epithelium）

图 16 - 8　前列腺：人（HE 染色，×100）

Pic. 16 - 8　Prostate：Human. HE staining　×100

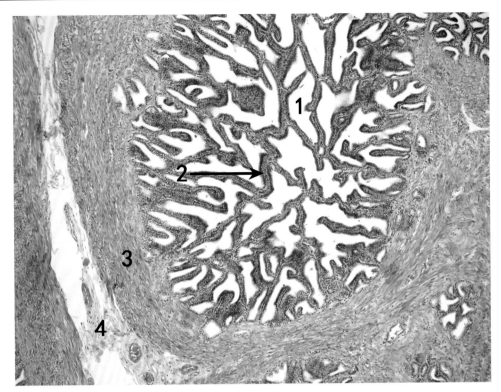

1.腺腔(gland cavity)　2.黏膜皱襞(mucosal fold)　3.肌层(muscularis)　4.外膜(adventitia)

图 16 - 9　精囊：人(HE 染色，×10)

Pic. 16 - 9　Seminal vesicle：Human. HE staining　×10

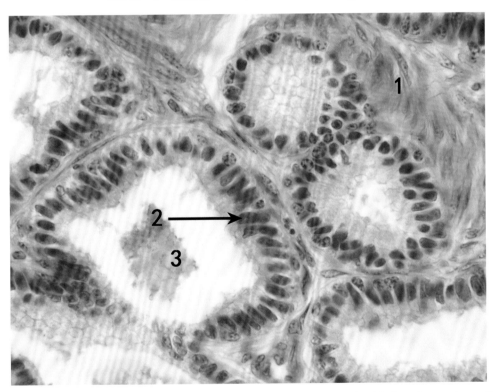

1.肌层的平滑肌(rich smooth muscle fibers in muscularis)　2.黏膜的假复层柱状上皮(pseudostratified columnar epithelium of mucosa)　3.腺腔(acinus)

图 16 - 10　精囊黏膜：人(HE 染色，×100)

Pic. 16 - 10　Mucosa of seminal vesicle：Human. HE staining　×100

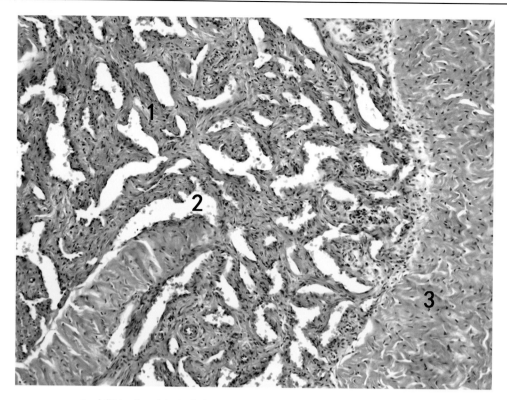

1. 小梁（trabecula） 2. 血窦（vascular space） 3. 白膜（tunica albuginea）

图 16 - 11　阴茎海绵体：人（HE 染色，×10）

Pic. 16 - 11　Corpus cavernosum of penis：Human. HE staining　×10

第十七章　女性生殖系统

实验基本要求：

1. 了解女性生殖系统的组成和功能。

2. 了解卵巢的一般结构。掌握原始卵泡、初级卵泡、次级卵泡和成熟卵泡的形态结构。黄体、闭锁卵泡和间质腺的形态、结构和功能。

3. 了解阴道和乳腺的结构特点。

4. 熟悉输卵管的结构与功能。

5. 掌握子宫壁和子宫颈的一般结构和周期性变化。

6. 光镜下识别卵巢、黄体、月经周期中各期子宫和阴道。

7. 相关超微结构和功能可通过课堂讨论等完成。

Chapter 17　Female reproductive system

 Basic requirements for the experiment

1. Know the compositions and functions of female reproductive system.

2. Know the general structures of ovary. Master the morphology and structures of primordial, primary, secondary and mature follicle. The morphology, structures and functions of corpus luteum, atretic follicle and interstitial gland.

3. Know the structural features of vagina and mammary gland.

4. Familiar with the structures and functions of oviduct.

5. Master the general structures and periodic changing of uterus and cervix.

6. Identify ovary, oviduct, uterus in different phases of menstrual cycle and vagina under LM.

7. The corresponding EM structures and functions will be discussed in lab.

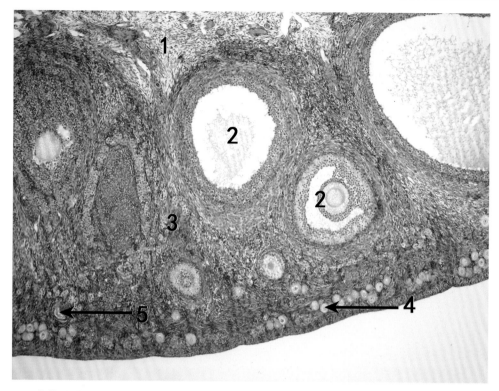

1.卵巢髓质(ovarian medulla) 2.次级卵泡(secondary follicle) 3.卵巢皮质(ovarian cortex)

4.原始卵泡(primordial follicle) 5.闭锁卵泡(atretic follicle)

图 17 - 1　卵巢：兔(HE 染色，×10)

Pic. 17 - 1　Ovary：Rabbit. HE staining　×10

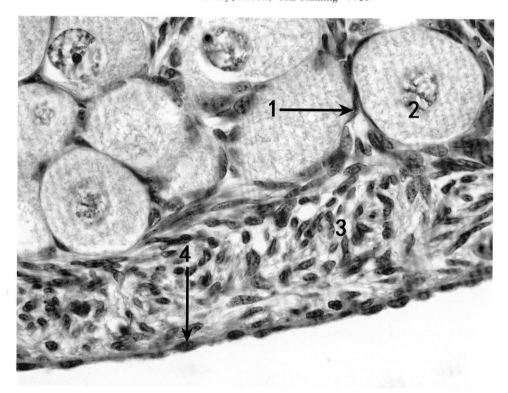

1.卵泡细胞(follicular cell) 2.初级卵母细胞(primary oocyte) 3.白膜(tunica albuginea)

4.表面上皮(superficial epithelium)

图 17 - 2　原始卵泡：兔(HE 染色，×100)

Pic. 17 - 2　Primordial follicle：Rabbit. HE staining　×100

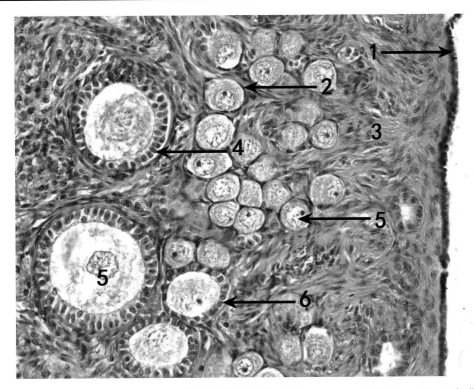

1. 表面上皮(superficial epithelium) 2. 单层扁平卵泡细胞(single squamous follicular cell) 3. 白膜(tunica albuginea) 4. 单层柱状卵泡细胞(single columnar follicular cell) 5. 初级卵母细胞(primary oocyte) 6. 单层立方卵泡细胞(single cuboidal follicular cell)

图 17-3 初级卵泡:兔(HE 染色,×40)

Pic. 17-3 Primary follicle:Rabbit. HE staining ×40

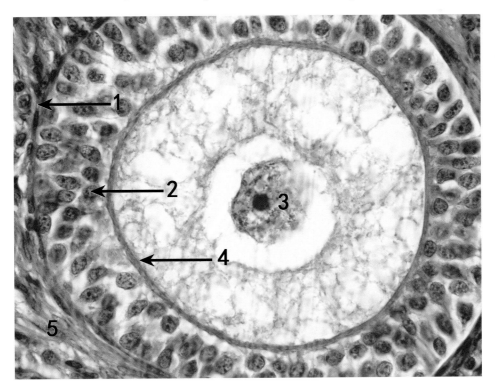

1. 基膜(basement membrane) 2. 卵泡细胞(follicular cell) 3. 初级卵母细胞的胞核(nucleus of primary oocyte)

4. 透明带(zona pellucida) 5. 卵泡膜(follicular theca)

图 17-4 初级卵泡:兔(HE 染色,×100)

Pic. 17-4 Primary follicle:Rabbit. HE staining ×100

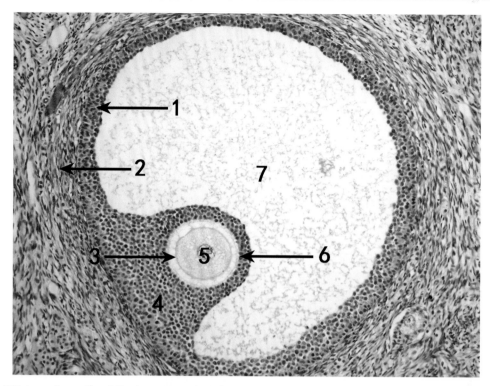

1.粒细胞(granulosa cell in follicular wall) 2.卵泡膜(follicular theca) 3.透明带(zona pellucida) 4.卵丘(cumulus oophorus) 5.初级卵母细胞(primary oocyte) 6.放射冠(corona radiata) 7.卵泡腔(follicular cavity)

图 17－5　次级卵泡：兔(HE 染色，×20)

Pic. 17－5　Secondary follicle：Rabbit. HE staining　×20

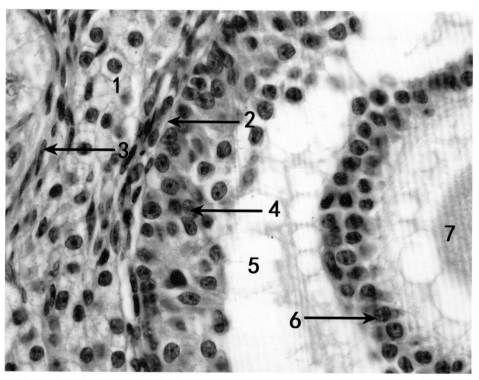

1.卵泡膜内层膜细胞(theca cell in theca interna) 2.基膜(basement membrane) 3.卵泡膜外层(theca externa) 4.卵泡壁粒细胞(granulosa cells in follicular wall) 5.卵泡腔(follicular cavity) 6.放射冠(corona radiata) 7.初级卵母细胞(primary oocyte)

图 17－6　次级卵泡：兔(HE 染色，×100)

Pic. 17－6　Secondary follicle：Rabbit. HE staining　×100

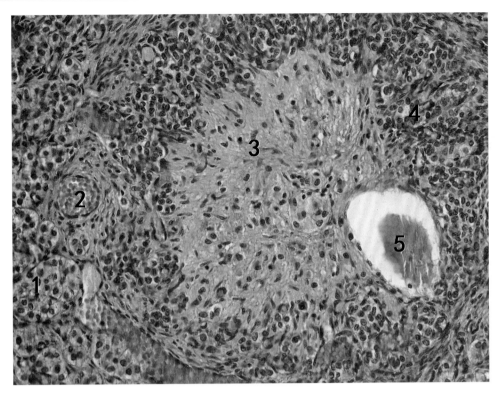

1. 间质腺（interstitial gland）2. 小血管（small blood vessel）3. 增生的结缔组织（proliferating connective tissue）
4. 退化的粒细胞（atretic granulosa cell）5. 退化的透明带和卵母细胞（atretic zona pellucida and oocyte）

图 17 - 7　闭锁卵泡：兔（HE 染色，×40）

Pic. 17 - 7　Atretic follicle：Rabbit. HE staining　×40

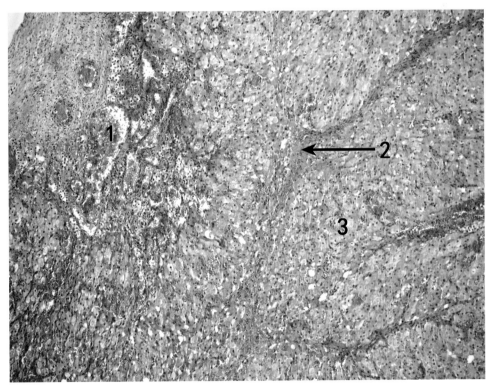

1. 小血管（small blood vessel）2. 黄体组织（corpus luteum tissue）3. 结缔组织隔（connective tissue septum）

图 17 - 8　黄体：兔（HE 染色，×40）

Pic. 17 - 8　Corpus luteum：Rabbit. HE staining　×40

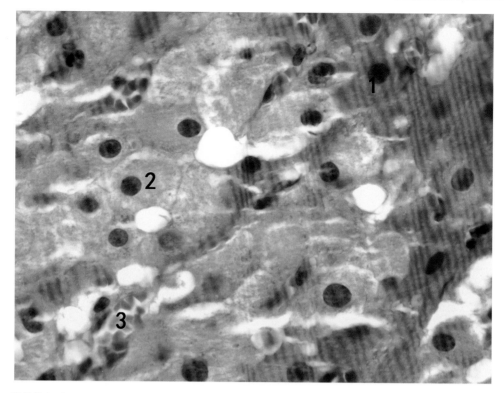

1.膜黄体细胞（theca lutein cell） 2.颗粒黄体细胞（granulosa lutein cell） 3.小血管（small blood vessel）

图 17 - 9　黄体：兔（HE 染色，×100）

Pic. 17 - 9　Corpus luteum：Rabbit. HE staining　×100

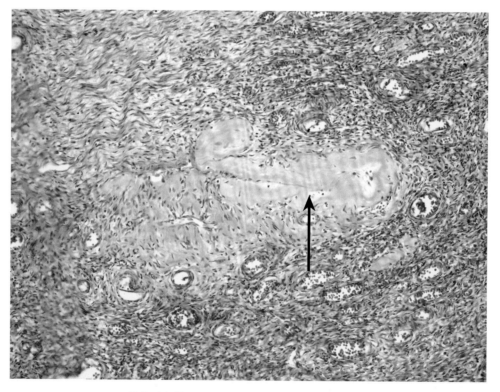

箭头示白体。The arrow shows corpus albicans.

图 17 - 10　白体：兔（HE 染色，×20）

Pic. 17 - 10　Corpus albicans：Rabbit. HE staining　×20

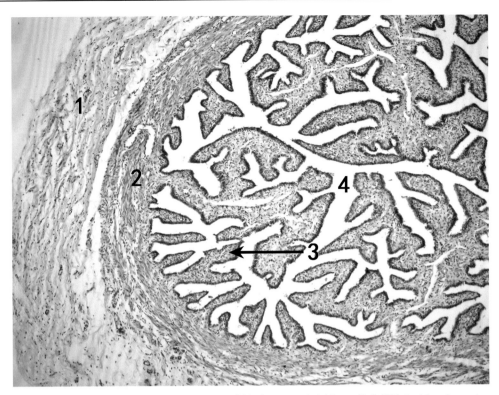

1.浆膜(serosa) 2.肌层(muscularis) 3.黏膜皱襞(mucosal fold) 4.输卵管腔(oviduct lumen)

图 17 - 11 输卵管:人(HE 染色,×10)

Pic. 17 - 11 Oviduct:Human. HE staining ×10

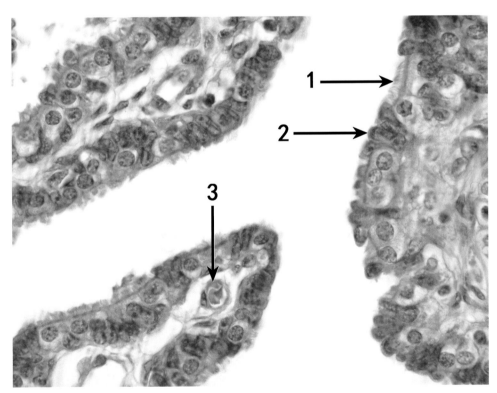

1.黏膜上皮纤毛细胞(ciliated cells of mucosal epithelium) 2.黏膜上皮分泌细胞(secretory cell of mucosal epithelium)

3.黏膜固有层毛细血管(capillary in lamina propria)

图 17 - 12 输卵管黏膜:人(HE 染色,×100)

Pic. 17 - 12 Oviduct mucosa:Human. HE staining ×100

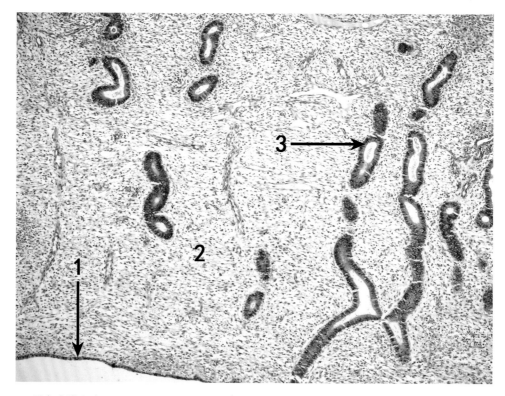

1. 子宫内膜上皮(endometrial epithelium) 2. 固有层(lamina propria) 3. 子宫腺(uterine gland)

图 17 - 13 增生期子宫内膜：人(HE 染色，×10)

Pic. 17 - 13 Endometrium of proliferative phase：Human. HE staining ×10

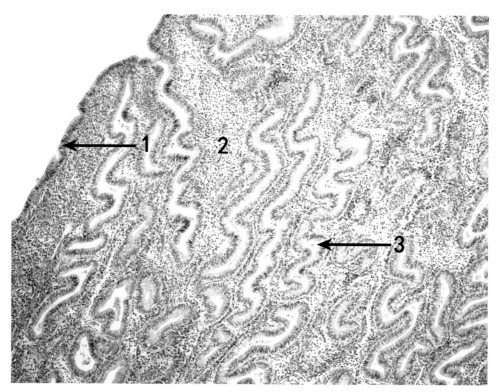

1. 子宫内膜上皮(endometrial epithelium) 2. 固有层(lamina propria) 3. 子宫腺(uterine gland)

图 17 - 14 分泌期子宫内膜：人(HE 染色，×10)

Pic. 17 - 14 Endometrium of secretory phase：Human. HE staining ×10

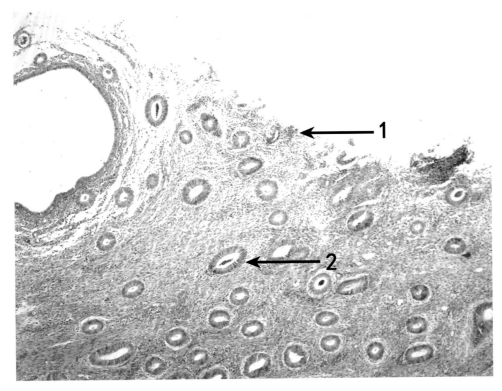

1.剥落的黏膜组织(shedding endometrium)　2.子宫腺(uterine gland)

图 17 - 15　月经期子宫内膜:人(HE 染色,×10)

Pic. 17 - 15　Endometrium of menstrual phase:Human. HE staining　×10

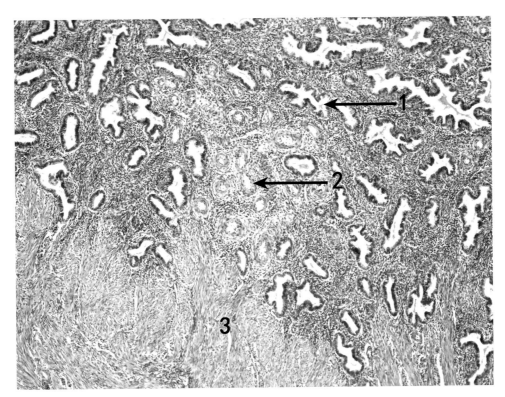

1.分泌期子宫内膜的子宫腺(uterine gland in endometrium of secretory phase)　2.螺旋动脉(spiral artery)

3.子宫肌层(myometrium)

图 17 - 16　螺旋动脉:人(HE 染色,×10)

Pic. 17 - 16　Spiral artery:Human. HE staining　×10

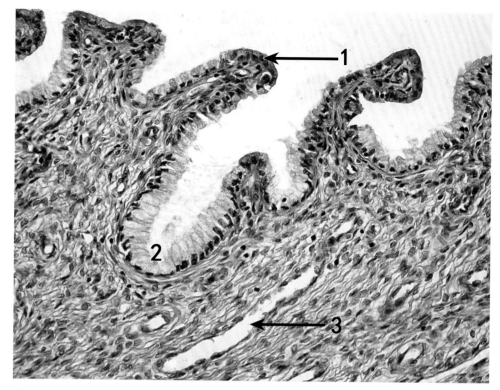

1. 子宫颈黏膜单层柱状上皮（simple columnar epithelium of cervical mucosa） 2. 子宫颈腺（cervical gland）

3. 小血管（small blood vessel）

图 17 - 17　子宫颈：人（HE 染色，×40）

Pic. 17 - 17　Cervix：Human. HE staining　×40

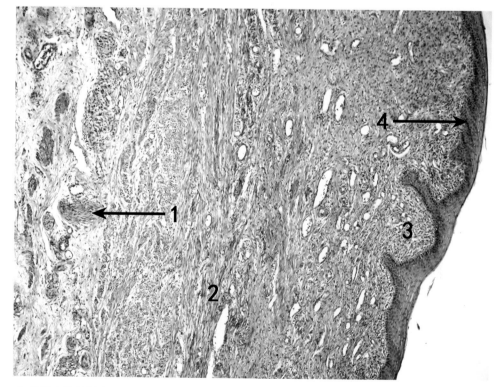

1. 外膜中的神经束（nerve bundle in adventitia） 2. 肌层（muscularis） 3. 固有层（lamina propria）

4. 黏膜上皮/复层扁平上皮（mucosal epithelium/stratified squamous epithelium）

图 17 - 18　阴道：人（HE 染色，×10）

Pic. 17 - 18　Vagina：Human. HE staining　×10

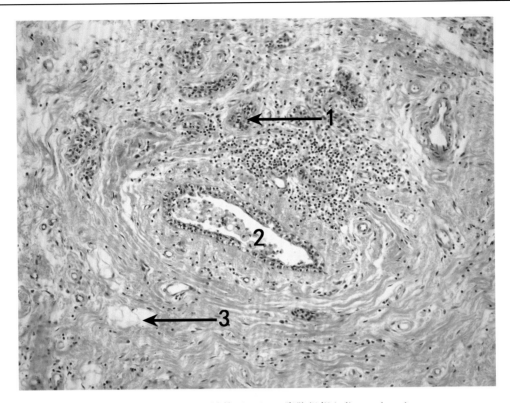

1.腺泡(alveolus) 2.导管(duct),3.脂肪组织(adipose tissue)

图 17 - 19 静止期乳腺:猫(HE 染色,×10)

Pic. 17 - 19 Inactive mammary gland:Cat. HE staining ×10

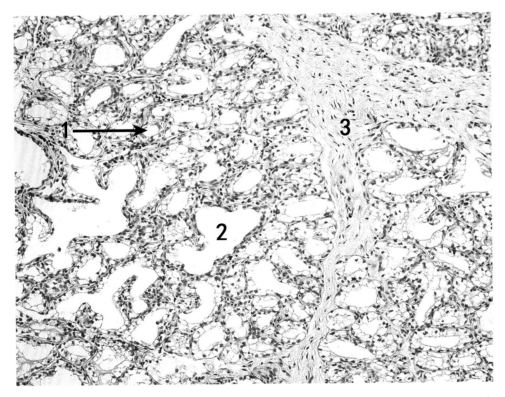

1.腺泡(alveolus) 2.小叶内导管(intralobular duct) 3.结缔组织间隔(connective tissue septum)

图 17 - 20 活动期乳腺:猫(HE 染色,×10)

Pic. 17 - 20 Active mammary gland:Cat. HE staining ×10

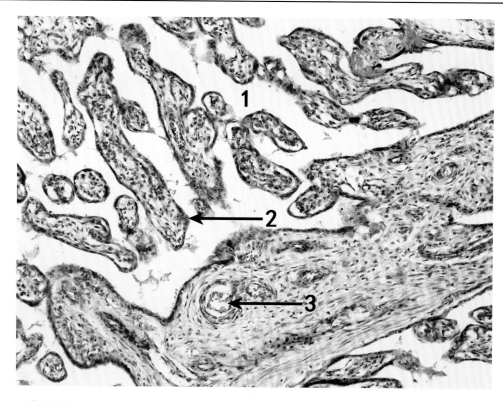

1. 绒毛间隙(intervillous space) 2. 绒毛表面的滋养层细胞(trophoblastic cells on villous surface)

3. 干绒毛内的小血管(small blood vessel in a stem villus)

图 17 – 21 胎盘绒毛：人(HE 染色，×20)

Pic. 17 – 21 Placental villus：Human. HE staining ×20

第十八章　眼和耳

实验基本要求：

1. 了解眼的组成。熟悉视盘、晶状体、玻璃体、房水的组成、组织结构和功能。掌握角膜、巩膜、巩膜静脉窦、脉络膜、虹膜、前房、后房、睫状体、视网膜、色素上皮细胞、黄斑。

2. 了解耳的组成。熟悉壶腹嵴、位觉斑、蜗管和螺旋器的组织结构和功能。

3. 光镜下识别角膜、虹膜、睫状体、晶状体、视网膜、壶腹嵴和螺旋器。

4. 相关超微结构和功能可通过课堂讨论等完成。

Chapter 18　Eye and ear

 Basic requirements for the experiment

1. Know the compositions of eye. Familiar with optic disc, lens, vitreous body and aqueous humor. Master the compositions, structures and functions of cornea, sclera, scleral venous sinus, choroid, iris, anterior chamber, posterior chamber, ciliary body, retina, pigment epithelial cells, macula lutea.

2. Know the compositions of ear. Familiar with the structures and functions of crista ampullaris, macula staticae, cochlear duct and spiral organ.

3. Identify cornea, iris, ciliary body, lens, retina, crista ampullaris and spiral organ under LM.

4. The corresponding EM structures and functions will be discussed in lab.

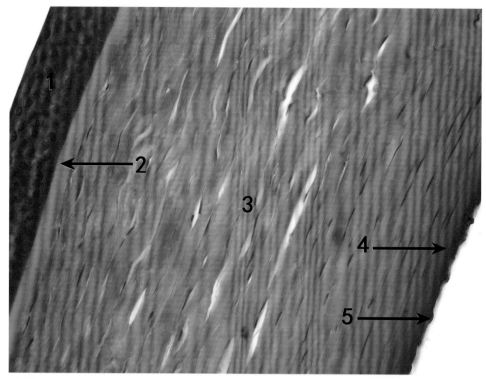

1.角膜上皮(corneal epithelium) 2.前界层(anterior limiting lamina) 3.角膜基质(corneal stroma)

4.后界层(posterior limiting lamina) 5.角膜内皮(corneal endothelium)

图 18-1　角膜:人(HE 染色,×40)

Pic. 18-1　Cornea:Human. HE staining　×40

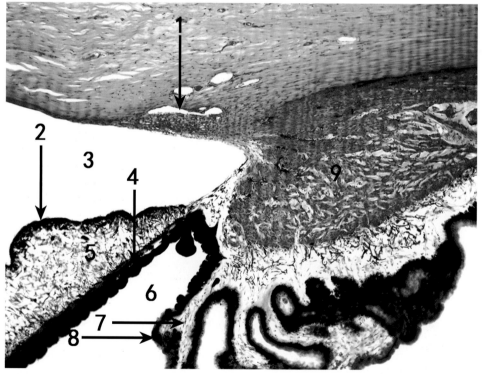

1.巩膜静脉窦(scleral venous sinus) 2.虹膜前缘层(anterior border layer of iris) 3.前房(anterior chamber)

4.虹膜上皮(iris epithelium) 5.虹膜基质(iris stroma) 6.后房(posterior chamber) 7.睫状突(ciliary process)

8.睫状体上皮(ciliary epithelium) 9.睫状肌(ciliary muscle)

图 18-2　眼前部:人(HE 染色,×10)

Pic. 18-2　Anterior part of eye:Human. HE staining　×10

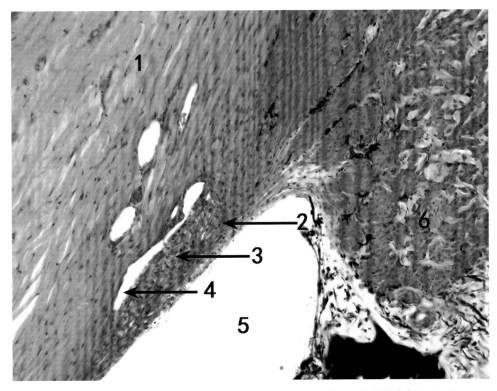

1. 巩膜(sclera)　2. 巩膜距(scleral spur)　3. 小梁网(trabecular meshwork)　4. 巩膜静脉窦(scleral venous sinus)

5. 后房(posterior chamber)　6. 睫状肌(ciliary muscle)

图 18 - 3　眼前部：人(HE 染色，×20)

Pic. 18 - 3　Anterior part of eye：Human. HE staining　×20

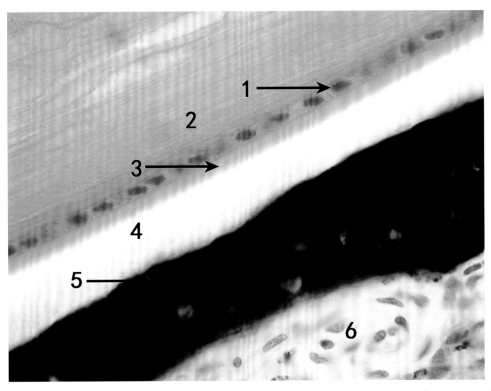

1. 晶状体上皮(lens epithelium)　2. 晶状体纤维(lens fibers)　3. 晶状体囊(lens capsule)　4. 后房(posterior chamber)

5. 虹膜上皮(iris epithelium)　6. 虹膜基质(iris stroma)

图 18 - 4　晶状体和虹膜：人(HE 染色，×100)

Pic. 18 - 4　Lens and iris：Human. HE staining　×100

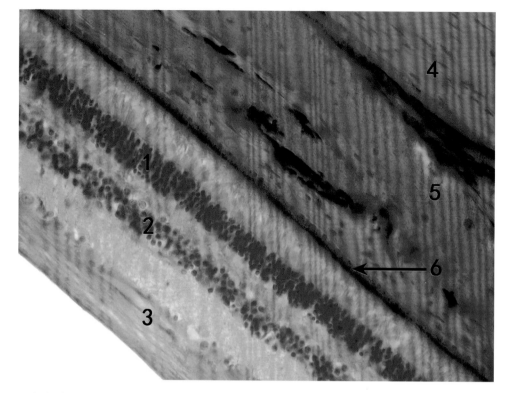

1. 视细胞(visual cells) 2. 中间神经元(interneurons) 3. 节细胞(ganglion cells) 4. 巩膜(sclera)
5. 脉络膜(choroid) 6. 色素上皮细胞(pigment epithelial cells)

图 18-5 视网膜视部和脉络膜：人(HE 染色，×40)

Pic. 18-5 Pars optica retina and choroid：Human. HE staining ×40

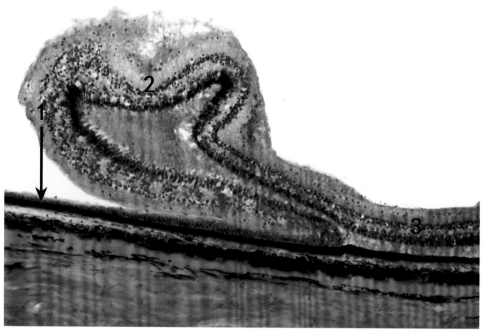

1. 视网膜盲部(pars caeca retina) 2. 锯齿缘(ora serrata) 3. 视网膜视部(pars optica retina)

图 18-6 视网膜盲部：人(HE 染色，×20)

Pic. 18-6 Pars caeca retina：Human. HE staining ×20

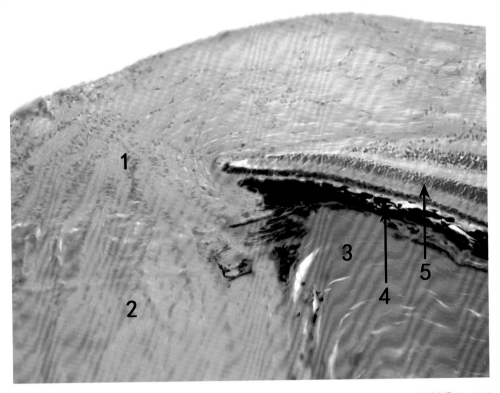

1.视盘（optic disc） 2.视神经（optic nerve） 3.巩膜（sclera） 4.脉络膜（choroid） 5.视网膜（retina）

图 18-7 视盘：人（HE 染色，×20）

Pic. 18-7 Optic disc：Human. HE staining ×20

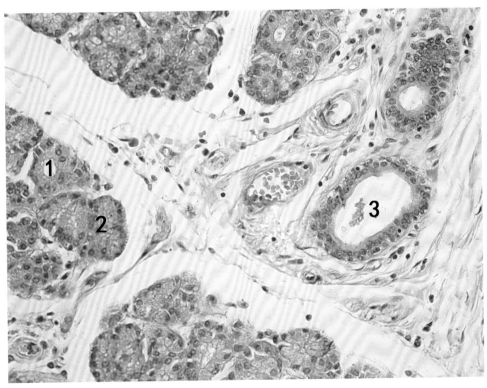

1.小叶内导管（intralobular duct） 2.浆液性腺泡（serous acinus） 3.小叶间导管（interlobular duct）

图 18-8 泪腺：人（HE 染色，×40）

Pic. 18-8 Lacrimal gland：Human. HE staining ×40

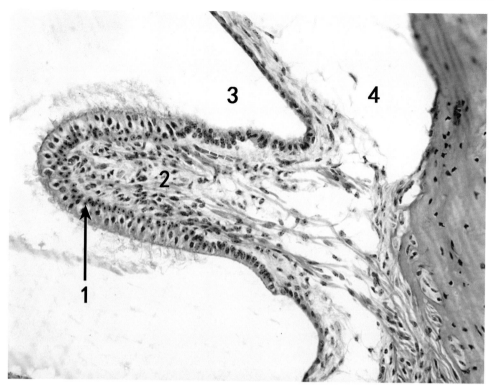

1.壶腹帽(cupula) 2.壶腹嵴(crista ampullaris) 3.膜半规管腔(lumen of membranous semicircular canal)

4.骨半规管腔(lumen of bony semicircular canal)

图 18 – 9　壶腹嵴:豚鼠(HE 染色,×20)

Pic. 18 – 9　Crista ampullaris:Guinea pig. HE staining　×20

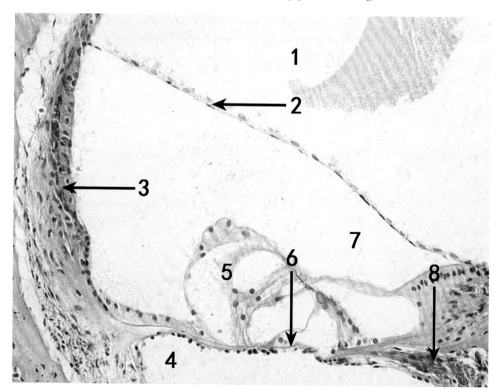

1.前庭阶(scala vestibuli) 2.前庭膜(vestibular membrane) 3.血管纹(stria vascularis) 4.鼓室阶(scala tympani)

5.螺旋器(spiral organ) 6.基底膜(basilar membrane) 7.蜗管(cochlear duct) 8.螺旋神经(cochlear nerve)

图 18 – 10　耳蜗:豚鼠(HE 染色,×40)

Pic. 18 – 10　Cochlea:Guinea pig. HE staining　×40

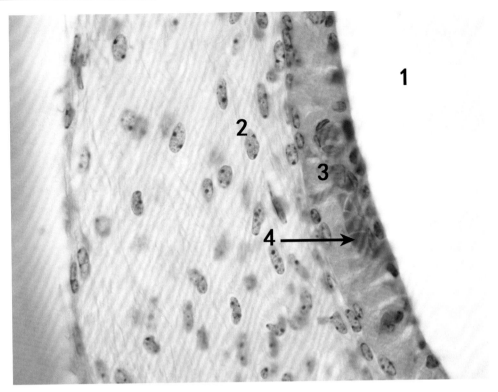

1.蜗管(cochlear duct)　2.螺旋韧带(spiral ligament)　3.血管纹(stria vascularis)　4.毛细血管(capillary)

图 18 - 11　血管纹:豚鼠(HE 染色,×100)

Pic. 18 - 11　Stria vascularis:Guinea pig. HE staining　×100

参 考 文 献

1. 石玉秀.组织学与胚胎学:3 版[M].北京:高等教育出版社,2018.
2. 石玉秀.组织学与胚胎学图谱:3 版[M].北京:高等教育出版社,2018.
3. 李和,李继承.组织学与胚胎学:3 版[M].北京:人民卫生出版社,2015.
4. 董为人,马保华,李和.人体组织学数字切片图谱[M].西安:西安交通大学出版社,2015.
5. Ronald W. Dudek,罗娜.医学组织学图谱[M].北京:人民卫生出版社,2013.
6. 周劲松.组织学与胚胎学[M].南京:江苏科学技术出版社,2013.

References

1. Yuxiu Shi. Histology and Embryology. 3rd edition[M]. Beijing:Higher Education Press. 2018.
2. Yuxiu Shi. Atlas of Histology and Embryology. 3rd edition[M]. Beijing:Higher Education Press. 2018.
3. He Li,Jicheng Li. Histology and Embryology. 3rd edition[M]. Beijing:People's Medical Publishing House. 2015.
4. Weiren Dong,Baohua Ma,He Li. Digital Atlas of Human Histology[M]. Xi'an: Xi'an Jiaotong University Press. 2015.
5. Ronald W D,Na Luo. Atlas of Medical Histology[M]. Beijing:People's Medical Publishing House. 2013.
6. Jinsong Zhou. Histology and Embryology[M]. Nanjing:Jiangsu Science and Technology Press. 2013.